CW00971085

the
perfume
Bible

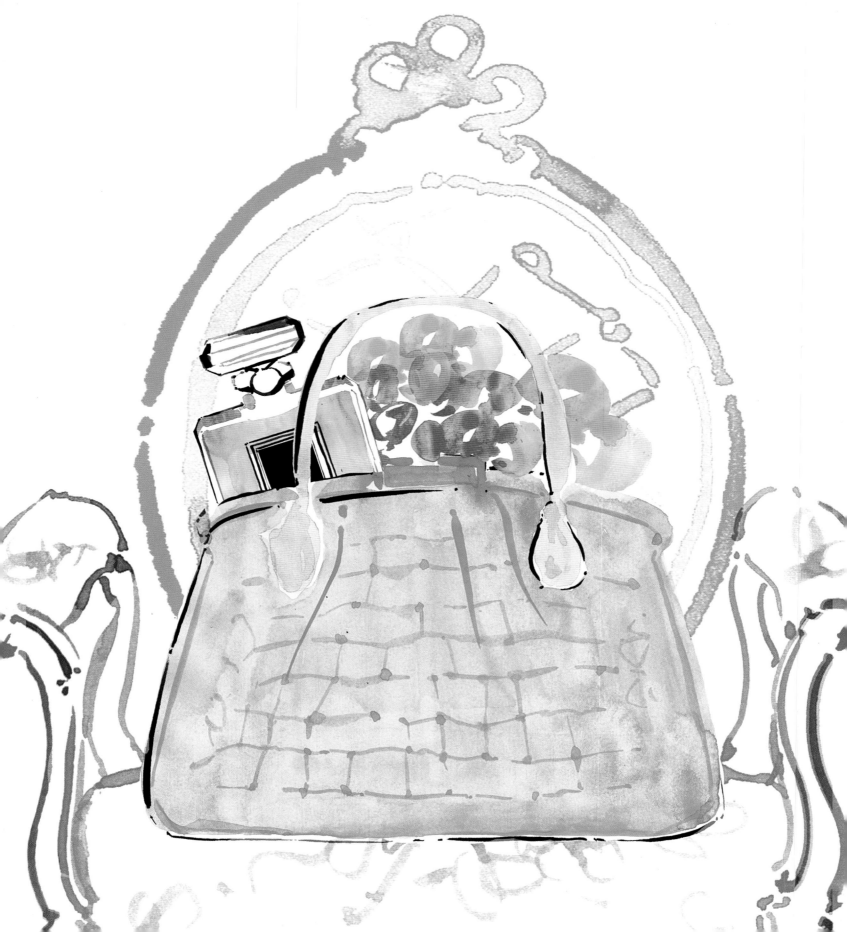

the perfume Bible

Josephine Fairley & Lorna McKay

Kyle Books

To Craig Sams and Nick McKay, who have been so supportive of us
on our perfumed adventure, with all our love

First published in Great Britain in 2014 by
Kyle Books
an imprint of Kyle Cathie Limited
192–198 Vauxhall Bridge Road
London SW1V 1DX
general.enquiries@kylebooks.com
www.kylebooks.com

10 9 8 7 6 5 4 3 2 1

ISBN: 978 0 85783 234 4

A CIP catalogue record for this title is available from the British Library

Josephine Fairley and Lorna McKay are hereby identified as the authors of this work in accordance with Section 77
of the Copyright, Designs and Patents Act 1988.

Fabric Credits
Issey Miyake L'Eau d'Issey - Sanderson Sparkle Coral Embroidery Silver/Aegean DAEG232977
Liz Earle Botanical Essence No. 15 - Romo, Mokoshi Eden V3039/03
Kenzo Flower by Kenzo - Villa Nova, Elodie Washable Carmine V3101/02

Editor: Vicky Orchard
Design: Jenny Semple
Photographer: Neal Grundy
Stylist: Charlie Davis
Illustrations: Kerrie Hess (www.kerriehess.com) apart from those listed on pages 190–191
Map illustration (pages 52–53): Alice Tait (www.alicetait.com)
Picture research: Vicky Orchard and Hannah Coughlin
Copy editor: Liz Murray
Production: Lisa Pinnell

Colour reproduction by ALTA London
Printed and bound in China by Toppan Leefung Printing Ltd

contents

introduction   6

meet the families   8

perfume portraits   14

from strength to strength   20

how to find your next scent love   26

do you speak perfume?   30

signature scent –v– a wardrobe of fragrances   36

how the magic of scent works on the mind   42

scents of time   46

a world of ingredients   52

what the noses know   56

from field to flacon: the making of a perfume   62

natural –v– synthetic   70

plant a perfume   72

collecting perfume art   76

perfume, bottled   80

collecting vintage perfume bottles   82

small(ish) is beautiful   84

a bespoke fragrance: the ultimate luxury   92

top 100 perfumes to try before you die   98

the men's room   148

(some of) the best perfume shops in the world   158

perfume and the blogosphere   162

everything you ever wanted to know about fragrance…   166

Directory   180

Index   183

introduction

The sense of smell, as Helen Keller put it, is 'the fallen angel of our senses'. We no longer need our noses to warn us of approaching sabre-toothed tigers, or to help us find our dinner in the hedgerows. Today, our noses operate at just a fraction of their capacity and, as a result, we're missing out on a huge pleasure quotient.

But we think all that's about to change, which is why we've written *The Perfume Bible*. Twenty years ago, chefs came out of the kitchens and inspired a new generation of food lovers to explore ingredients, stories, and to learn by experimenting and tasting. Today, something similar is happening in the world of fragrance. Perfumers, if you like, are 'the new chefs'. And this time, it's our nostrils that are getting all tingly and excited, not our taste buds.

This shift began when a man called Frederic Malle launched a collection of scents that not only had his name on the bottle, it proclaimed the name of the perfumer who'd created it. Frederic Malle's stroke of brilliance was to ask some of the leading perfumers in the world – who'd mostly been working quietly behind the scenes – to create the perfume they'd dreamed of – their 'perfect perfume', if you like. Those 'noses' were invited to come 'out of the closet' – out of the lab, in fact – and share their inspirations, in scent form.

The beauty press got excited. We shared it with readers, who got even more

Get a whisper of your mother's scent from a stranger walking by, and you're back in a dimly-lit bedroom, enveloped in love as she kisses you goodnight.

excited. And this kick-started a whole new era of creativity in the perfume world, with 'niche'/cult perfume start-ups now making their mark in every country and major fragrance houses 'upping their game' with rare and precious creations for us to lust after: Chanel with Les Exclusifs, Dior's La Collection Privée, Armani Privé... (Though don't run away with the idea this book's only about the scent equivalent of truffles and smoked salmon: there's plenty of 'everyday' gorgeousness in these pages.)

But the bottom line is that, as the veil of secrecy has fallen away from perfume, women (and men) who'd perhaps never given a thought to the story behind a scent, or its ingredients, have found themselves in a wonderland of fragrant discovery. It's like being invited to 'step through the back of the wardrobe', into the scent equivalent of Narnia.

All this has led to an explosion in the sheer number of fragrances being launched, as this area of the beauty world opens up. But there's a flip side: confusion. (And sensory overload, sometimes, as you dodge the 'guerilla sprayers' in a department store.) So as well as inviting you to explore the fascinating process behind creating a perfume, discover ingredients from around the world and meet some of the 'stars' of the scent world, we're also here to lead you by the hand – or maybe that should be the nose – through Narnia, to fragrances you'll love. Or which – simply because of their 'iconic' status – are worth sniffing out because they're important landmarks: the perfume world's equivalent of Monet's *Water Lilies*, or the *Mona Lisa*, or Rodin's *The Kiss*. The difference is: these are works of art you can actually take home and wear, every day (or night). They're not the museum shop 'repros': they're the real deal.

Why buy a book about perfume? Why not just go round smelling a bit more consciously? For a very good reason. When you start to put words to aromas, something truly extraordinary – miraculous, we'd call it – starts to happen. As our scientist friend Professor George Dodd (who set up the Olfaction Research Group at Warwick University) explains, 'You actually strengthen the neural pathways in the brain itself and, in turn, that helps you to become better at smelling things.' In other words, reading about perfumes and perfumery can actually deepen your enjoyment of the scented world and turbocharge your pleasure in the perfumes you wear.

So we want you to think of this book as a springboard, really. The start of a journey that will take you back through fragrance's history, and fast-forward you into a world in which contemporary alchemists (the noses) blend essences to create bewitching stories in scent form. The fact is, 'fallen angel' or not, nothing has the power to Tardis us through time and space like our sense

> ❝
> *These are works of art you can actually take home and wear every day*
> ❞

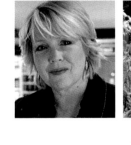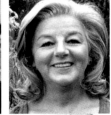

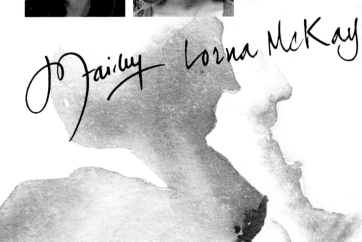

of smell. Get a whisper of your mother's scent from a stranger walking by and you're back in a dimly-lit bedroom, enveloped in love as she kisses you goodnight. (A cliché, maybe – but true for almost everyone we know.) Or walk into a room where a tomato leaf candle's flickering, perhaps – and suddenly you're in your grandma's greenhouse. Apply a touch of the perfume you wore for your wedding, and you're right there sharing your vows, all over again.

Wow. All that, from a little bottle, a spray or a spritz. If that isn't magic, we'd like to know what is…

meet the families

One of the easiest ways to start to explore perfume is by understanding that (almost) all fragrances fall into 'families'. What's more, funnily enough – and often without realising – it turns out that most women's successful fragrance purchases are roughly in the same 'family'. So if you want to save yourself from making expensive mistakes, it pays to know which fragrance family (or sometimes families) you belong to…

The fact is that one of the reasons women's dressing tables are often cluttered with perfume-shopping 'mistakes' is that – through responding to fabulous advertising imagery, or maybe being seduced by a 'celebrity' we like who has a new scent to sell – we may buy a fairly random collection of scents across different families, many of which we end up not really loving.

So a much, much more successful way to shop for fragrance is to explore other scents that belong to the same family as something you already wear and love. In reality, if an expert were to analyse our wardrobes of fragrances, very few of us have a mishmash of scents from across lots of different families: often without even realising, we do tend to fall for scents from one family time and again. Instinctively, we prefer scents from some fragrance families and dislike others – although we may tend towards one particular family for colder weather, another for sunny times. And there's no 'right or wrong' about what you're drawn to (we're almost violently anti-perfume snobbery); our fragrance preferences can be affected by our genes, our life experiences – and our memories.

Technically, fragrance families are a classification system the perfume industry has used for years to place individual perfumes into olfactory 'groups', based on their dominant characteristics. It's part of the language of scent. But it can feel baffling and complicated. So through the use of the colours on our Fragrance Fan, we aim to help you identify more easily – at a glance – which family the fragrances you already like fall into. Each fragrance in our Top 100 scents to try before you die is colour-coded (see pages 98–147); if you recognise something you like and wear, use the coding to seek out others in the same parent family.

A true family, of course, has lots of members – and so it is with fragrance. Most of the eight main fragrance families listed here have some variations on their theme.

It can certainly be helpful when you're fragrance shopping to know which family (or families) you're drawn to. If you're speaking to an informed sales consultant, they'll know which scents to steer you towards and you're more likely to find a new 'perfume love'.

In reality, only experts with years of experience can tell at first sniff which family a scent falls into: this takes practice. But the absolute very best way to learn these fragrance families is quite simply to use your nose…

PS Absolutely nobody in the perfume world agrees 100 per cent about families and descriptions. It's deeply frustrating. So we've used common sense and our years of knowledge and tried to simplify things as much as possible. Initially, if you want to learn more, try to become familiar with each of these main families. Then, as your nose develops, you can explore within those families and learn the nuances just as you would if you were learning about wine: first comes learning to tell a Chardonnay from a Sancerre. Over time you will be able to pick up the subtler differences within those types.

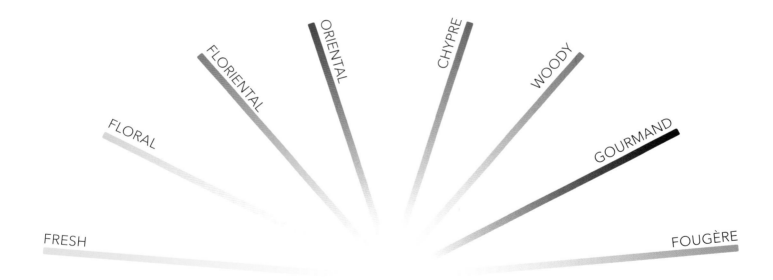

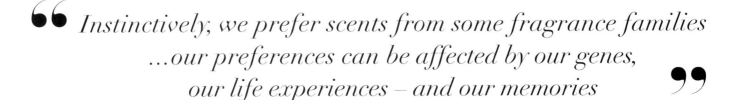

66 *Instinctively, we prefer scents from some fragrance families …our preferences can be affected by our genes, our life experiences – and our memories* 99

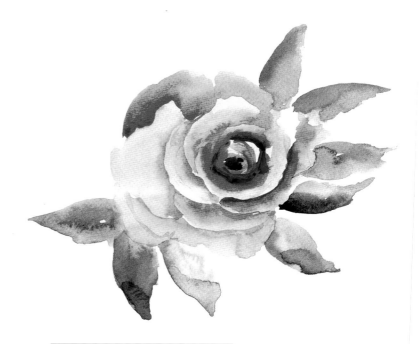

FRESH

Uplifting, zesty, cooling, most eaux de Cologne fall into this family. They feature a whoosh of notes such as lemon, bergamot, orange, grapefruit and mandarin. (These notes are also slightly randomly referred to as being 'hesperidic' – after the Hesperides, the nymphs from Greek mythology!) Fresh fragrances smell clean and usually come in the eau de toilette and Cologne versions – we can't think of a single 'fresh' scent in perfume concentration. Ideal for splashing, and probably more suited to summer, some conjure up a sea breeze while others smell like bottled sunshine. There are lots of 'near-relations' within the fresh category, so if you like your scents bright, uplifting, sunny and airy, spend some time sniffing and exploring.

Fresh fragrances include:

- Acqua di Parma Colonia by Acqua di Parma
- Ô de Lancôme by Lancôme
- Organic Glam Citron by The Organic Pharmacy
- Eau Universelle by L'Occitane

FLORAL

This is the most popular of all families with the vast majority of women's scents falling into this category. It's ultra-feminine (you won't find many unisex floral fragrances), and, of all the families, it's probably the one you'll most easily recognise at first sniff, from its bouquet of cut flowers conjuring up June weddings, garden parties, spring blossoms… Floral fragrances tend to be garlanded with notes such as jasmine, peony, gardenia, tuberose, lily of the valley, magnolia, mimosa, etc.

Interestingly, two of the most famous (and most-loved) floral notes – jasmine and rose – have traditionally been found at the heart of almost every fragrance creation: they're the perfume world's foundation stones. In true floral fragrances, those notes are played up – but shimmering beneath the surface of other families, rose and jasmine are often there, too, holding the creation together even when you can't spot them.

Florals can be warmed with a touch of spice or given the juiciness of fruits – and there are quite a few 'sub-families' in the floral family. (The 'floriental' family is a close cousin, too.) If you veer towards florals, you will never be bored: there's an endless abundance of flora to explore.

Florals include:

- White Gardenia Petals by Illuminum
- Very Hollywood by Michael Kors
- Moschino Cheap & Chic by Moschino
- Live in Love by Oscar de la Renta

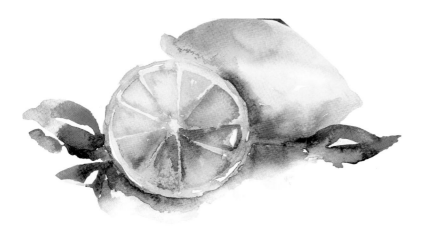

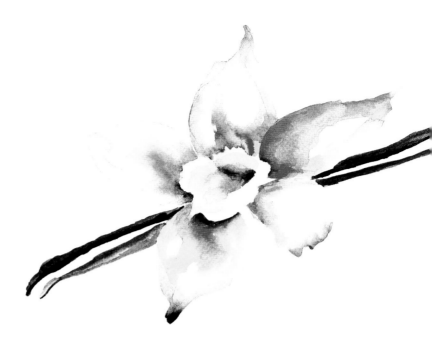

FLORIENTAL

The name says it all: the florientals are a sophisticated fusion of floral and Oriental notes and so many fragrances now fall into this category that it's a real family in its own right. Florientals blend flowers – including gardenia, jasmine, freesia and orange flower – with spices, warm woods and resins. The result? Fragrances that are sensual and often sweetly seductive, but generally airier and lighter than true Orientals. This family is growing incredibly fast, with fragrances that beef up the spiciness, the woodiness, or the fruits.

Floriental fragrances include:

- Chloé by Chloé
- Emporio Armani Diamonds by Armani
- Lady Million by Paco Rabanne
- The One by Dolce & Gabbana

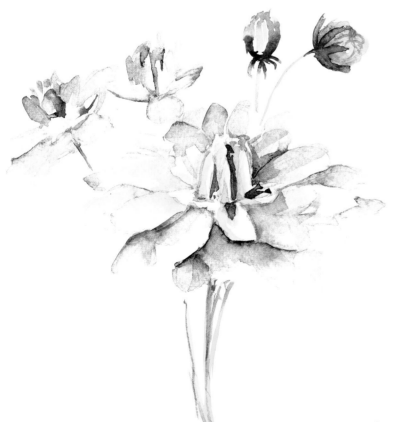

ORIENTAL

With their spices, musks, incense and resins, the Orientals are rooted in perfume's own history, using many of the same ingredients today that were first enjoyed in the Orient – in India and Arabia – at the dawn of fragrance creation.

Ingredients such as heliotrope, sandalwood, coumarin, orris, vanilla and gum resins are classically used within an Oriental fragrance structure – although these can be tweaked for men and women (and fragrances designed to be 'shared').

Seductive, voluptuous and with a va-va-voom, Orientals tend to feel 'grown-up' and many have a warm, heavy, diffusive richness that's more suited to after-dark wearing. They linger sensually on the skin: they're heavy on the base notes, which tend to last longer. (However, there is a new 'mini-family' of fresher Orientals, with a lighter touch and a more 'daytime' feel such as Chanel Coco Noir and Liz Earle Botanical Essence No.15.)

Oriental fragrances include:

- Shalimar by Guerlain
- Coco by Chanel
- Obsession by Calvin Klein
- Hammam Bouquet by Penhaligon's

GOURMAND

This is the newest family in the fragrance universe: the first blockbuster example was Thierry Mugler's Angel, and since then 'edible' notes have become super-popular. Think: caramel, chocolate, milk, candyfloss, coffee, Cognac, toffee, almonds, even bubblegum, and, almost always, a generous helping of vanilla. There may be spices in there, too, or amber: in general, gourmand fragrances are warm and most wearable in the cooler seasons, when we want a fragrance to snuggle up to.

Gourmand fragrances include:

- Angel by Thierry Mugler
- Prada Candy by Prada
- Tobacco Vanille by Tom Ford
- Lolita Lempicka by Lolita Lempicka

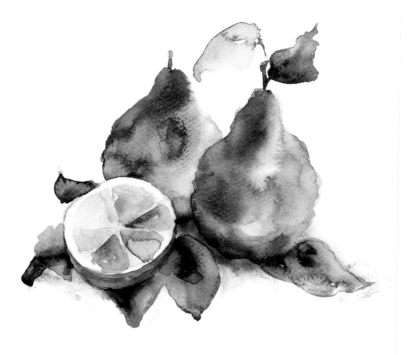

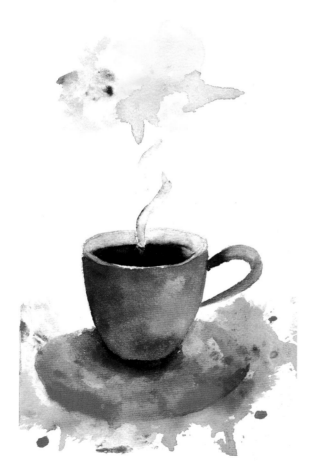

CHYPRE

First, how to say it: 'sheep-ra'. (From the French for Cyprus – not, as is often suggested, the cypress tree; Cyprus was the birthplace of Aphrodite, goddess of love and many aromatic perfume ingredients flourish there.) There are suggestions that chypre fragrance construction dates back to Roman times but it was certainly popularised by pioneering perfumer François Coty, who launched a ground-breaking scent called Chypre in 1917, and set feminine perfumery on a whole new, sophisticated course.

Chypre fragrances are warm and dry and almost all built around a woody, mossy accord of bergamot, oakmoss, patchouli and labdanum (from the cistus, or 'rock rose', plant). Elements of flowers, fruits or woodiness are sometimes played up in chypre fragrances – so this family has a few 'relations' within it.

Chypre fragrances include:

- No. 19 by Chanel
- Miss Dior by Dior
- Fiori di Capri by Carthusia
- Empreinte by Courrèges

WOODY

The clue, quite simply, is in the name – although some of these fragrances do smell like they're closely related to the chypre family. In fact, they share some characteristics, but generally without the floral flourishes of the chypres.

Perfumers have a fabulous palette of woody elements to weave into their creations: sandalwood, cedar, agarwood (aka oudh), guaiac wood (say it 'guy-ack'), as well as patchouli and vetiver. (These last two aren't woods: they're leaves and roots, respectively, but you'd never guess from their intensely earthy, woody characters.)

Woody fragrances can be given a spin by adding spices/fruity notes, or herbs – so if you like woods (or you're simply interested in learning what they smell like), there are plenty of variations to explore. Many masculine, quite a few shared and a few women's fragrances belong to the woody family.

Woody fragrances include:

- Sycomore by Chanel
- Vol de Nuit by Guerlain
- Rogart by Molton Brown
- Dzing! by L'Artisan Parfumeur

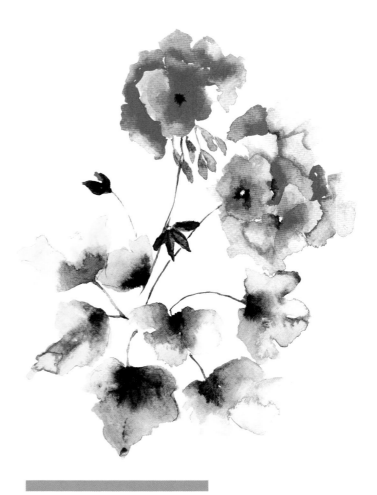

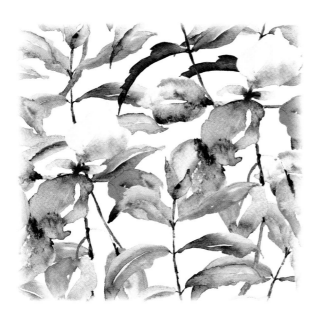

FOUGÈRE

Nowadays, it's mostly fragrances for men you'll find in the fougère category, which almost invariably features lavender, geranium, vetiver, bergamot, oakmoss and coumarin in the blend. It's a bit ironic, though, as this fragrance family was originally created for women, kicking off with Fougère Royale, from Houbigant, in 1882. Fougère takes its name from the French for 'fern' – and for anyone who's wondering, you say it 'foo-jair' (with the 'j' a little soft – almost 'foo-shair'). And if you'd like to start to understand what these ferny, green fragrances smell like, here are some classic examples to 'sniff out'.

Fougère fragrances include:

- Prada Pour Homme by Prada
- Joop! Homme by Joop
- Cerruti 1881 by Cerruti
- Suffolk Lavender by Shay & Blue

perfume portraits

The sheer number of fragrances out there – dozens of old faithfuls and non-stop new versions – can be nose-boggling.

And with more than 1,300 scents launched each year, how are we to find our perfect match? Well, it may be possible to take a shortcut to scents you're going to love through visual imagery: 'portraits', designed (like fragrance itself) to go straight for the emotions. This helps you to 'see', rather than guess, which scents suit you.

Follow your eyes, then find out (overleaf) which family the 'portraits' link you to – and read more, in meet the famillies (see pages 8–13). NB You may find yourself drawn to more than one montage – and that's fine; many of us like to match a fragrance to our differing moods…

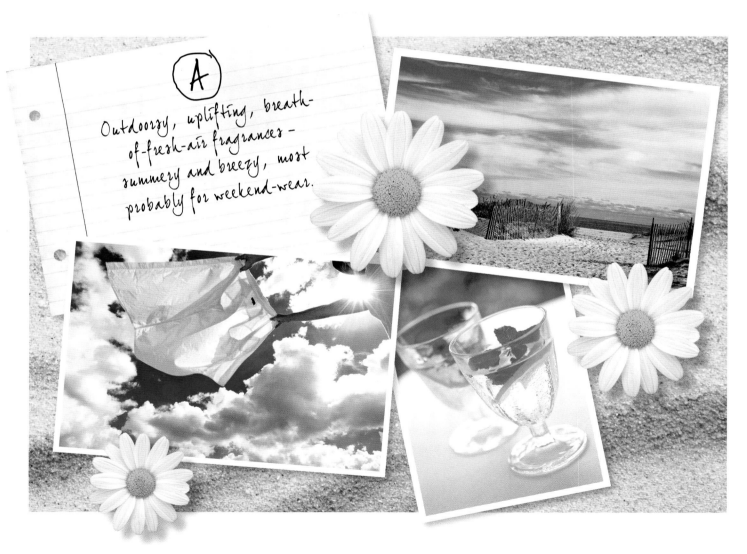

(A) *Outdoorzy, uplifting, breath-of-fresh-air fragrances – summery and breezy, most probably for weekend-wear.*

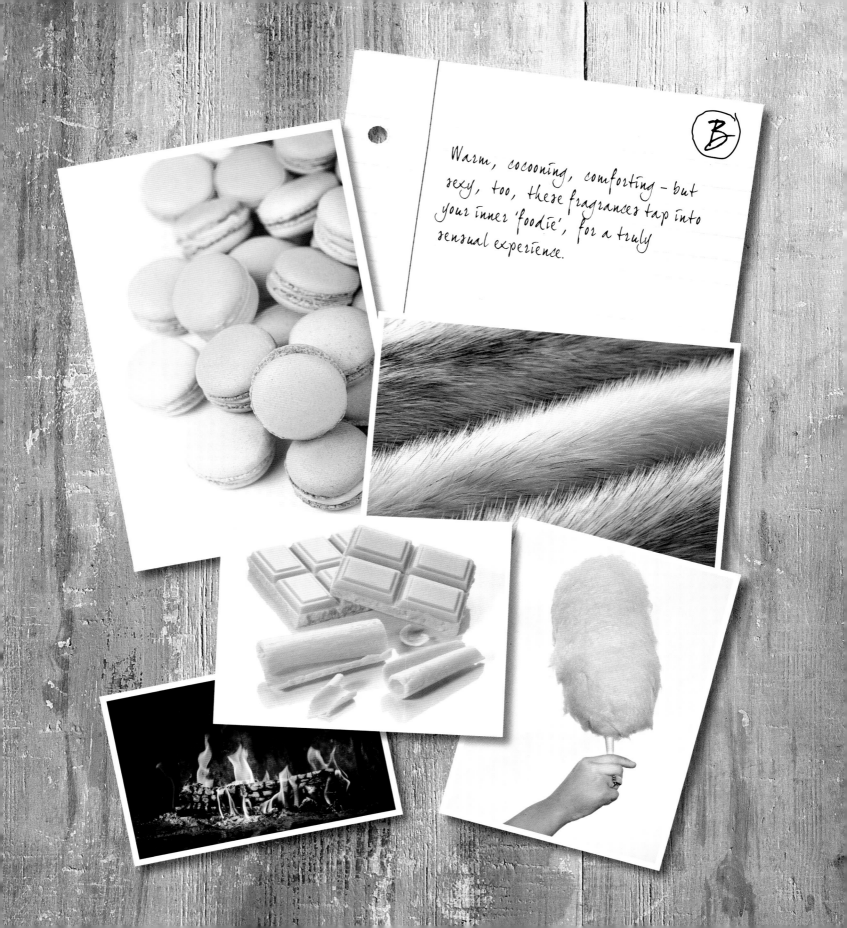

Warm, cocooning, comforting — but
sexy, too, these fragrances tap into
your inner 'foodie', for a truly
sensual experience.

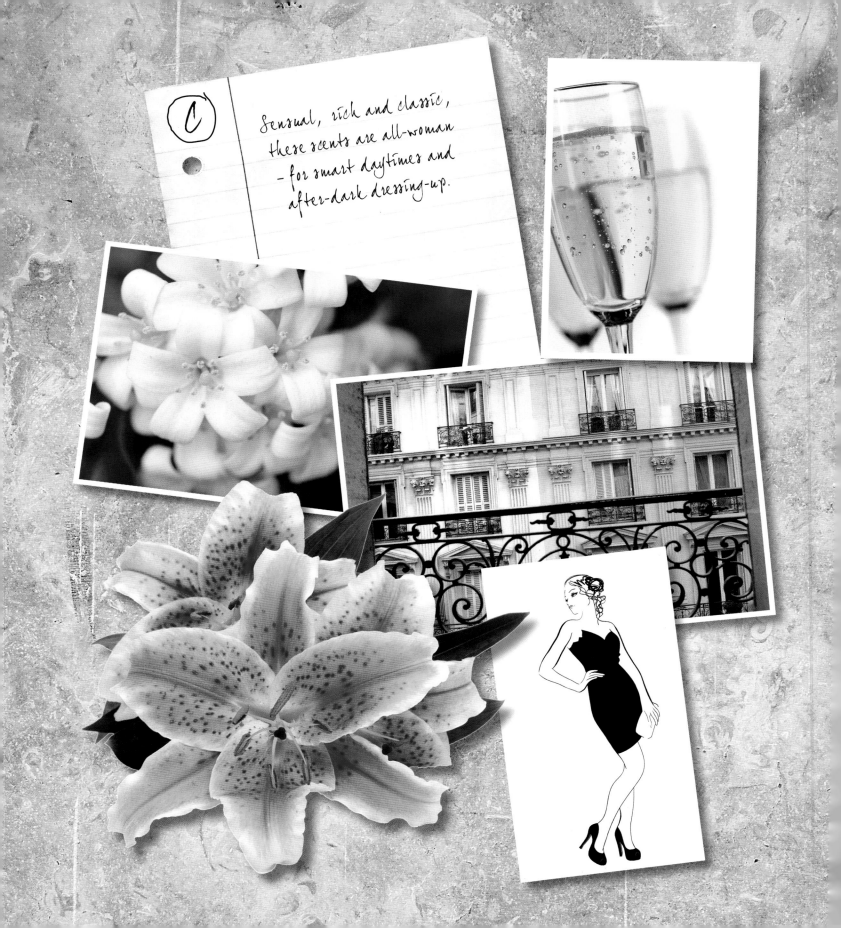

C

Sensual, rich and classic, these scents are all-woman – for smart daytimes and after-dark dressing-up.

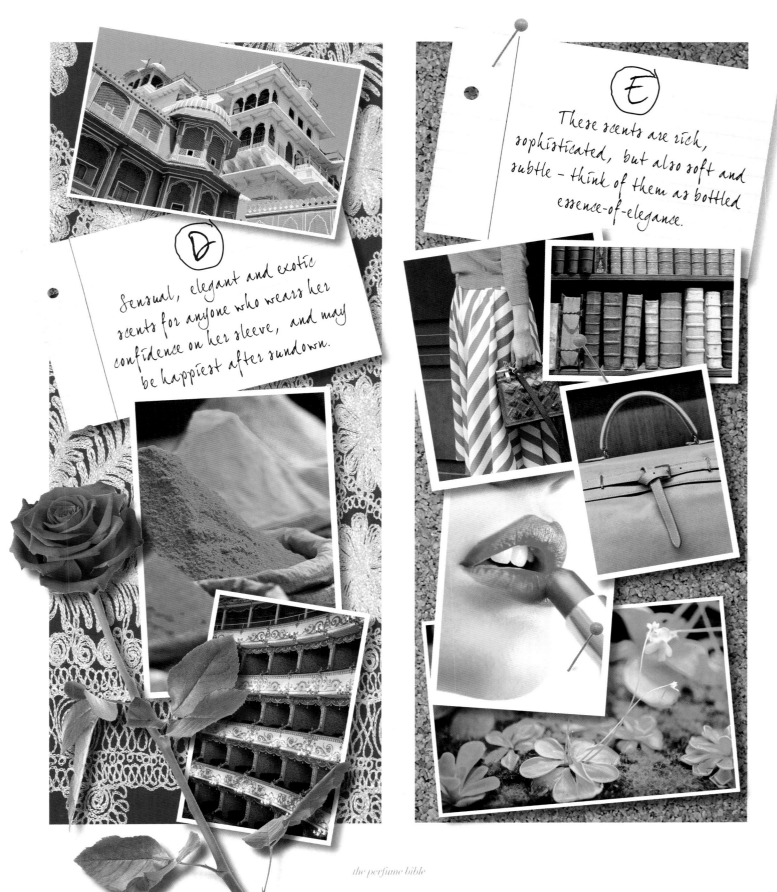

E

These scents are rich, sophisticated, but also soft and subtle – think of them as bottled essence-of-elegance.

D

Sensual, elegant and exotic scents for anyone who wears her confidence on her sleeve, and may be happiest after sundown.

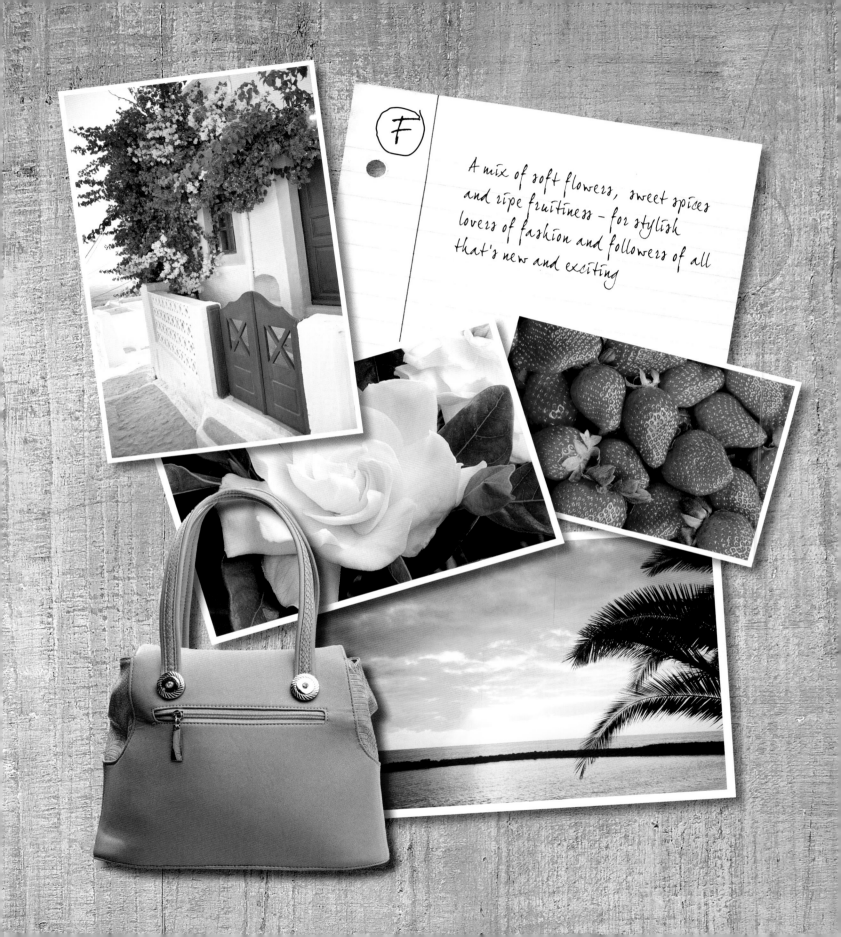

F

A mix of soft flowers, sweet spices
and ripe fruitiness - for stylish
lovers of fashion and followers of all
that's new and exciting

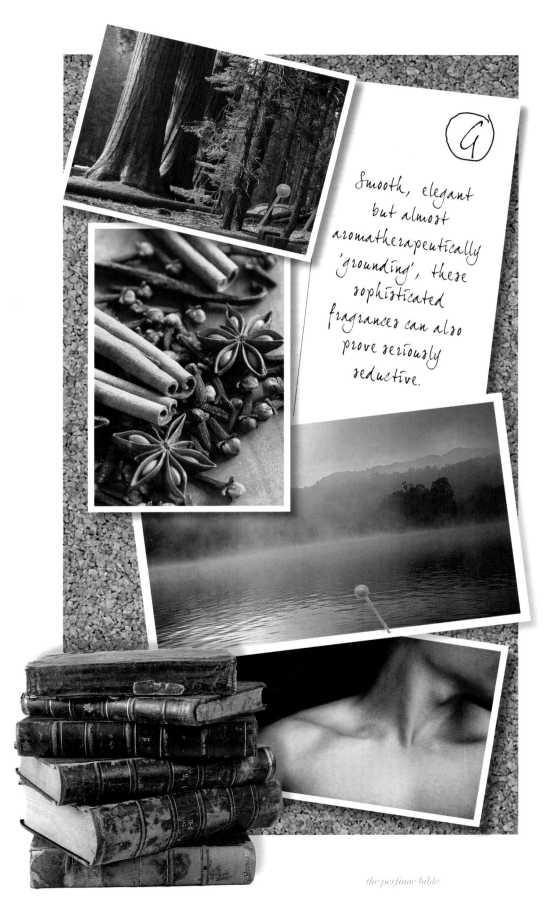

Smooth, elegant but almost aromatherapeutically 'grounding', these sophisticated fragrances can also prove seriously seductive.

Perfumers working on a brief are often given a visual representation by a perfume house of the mood and spirit they want a scent to evoke – so the use of imagery in fragrance creation is widespread. This follows the same principle. At-a-glance 'perfume portraits' can be effective because, according to perfume expert Dr Luca Turin:

"Scent is actually about much more than our sense of smell; it brings together all the senses"

Picture this

The montages you've just seen quickly conjure up different families, which you can read more about on pages 8–13, with some classic examples.

A. Fresh
B. Gourmand
C. Flora
D. Oriental
E. Chypre
F. Floriental
G. Woody

from STRENGTH *to* strength

As if shopping for fragrance wasn't confusing enough – you really aren't the first person to stand dithering at a crowded shelf of celebrity scents, classics and 'niche' perfumes, before walking away empty-handed – there's the 'strength' of these precious liquids to consider, too

You may already know that a bottle of (say) Chanel No. 5 parfum smells much more intense, and lasts longer, than the 'matching' eau de toilette – but your choice should reflect when (and how) you want to wear your scent…

How long your fragrance lasts on the skin is down to three factors. First, your skin type: fragrance 'dissipates' sooner on drier skins, but hangs around for longer on oilier complexions. (Possibly one of the few upsides of having shine-prone skin.) Second, the types of ingredients used: citrus notes are more 'volatile' and disappear sooner than smouldering spices, sexy musks and quietly humming woods.

But the third key factor is perfume 'strength'. And before you splash out – and splash on – you need to understand what's what. The basic rule of thumb is that the higher the concentration, or 'strength', the higher the price tag. But with the fairly recent arrival of many new, limited-distribution (and exciting) brands to shake up the perfume world, the rules on price no longer apply: some fairly 'light' fragrances nonetheless command some pretty hefty prices.

First things first: perfumes are essentially a mix of alcohol (ethanol), water and scented oils, or, in some cases, just ethanol and those precious oils.

Perfume or parfum – also sometimes referred to as 'pure perfume', 'perfume extract' or 'extrait de parfum' – features somewhere between 20–40 per cent of scented perfume ingredients, along with alcohol and/or water. According to the International Fragrance Association, or IFRA, the typical percentage is at the lower end – but this nevertheless intense concentration explains why the 'perfume' version of any fragrance is always the most expensive within a

Eau de toilette is the bestselling scent strength in the UK and many other countries

TIP

Heat is what activates perfume…

… specifically, body heat: the pulse points on your body (where your heartbeat can more easily be felt) are said to be the ideal places to apply a scent, as the skin is a tiny bit warmer there. Pulse points include the base of the throat, between the breasts, the wrists, the inside of the elbow and behind the knees, even just beside the ankle bone. But truly? We like Coco Chanel's advice. 'Where should one use perfume?' a young woman asked her. 'Wherever one wants to be kissed…' was Chanel's reply.

range. Perfumes/parfums (whatever you like to call them) are generally the longest-lasting on the skin – up to six or eight hours (and sometimes well into the next day) – with the best 'sillage': a wonderful word for how a fragrance projects before you, or trails behind you. Parfum is really for after-dark, for special occasions – weddings, parties – rather than for everyday; accordingly, these true 'perfumes' are often available in glass-stoppered bottles for dabbing, rather than the sprays and spritzers that lower concentrations tend to come in – making for a so-pleasurable ritual as you apply the pricy 'juice'.

Eau de parfum (which is also referred to as EDP) features a 10–20 per cent concentration of oils (typically somewhere around 15 per cent of those aromatic compounds). Again, these have lots of 'waft'; staying power of anywhere from 4–5 hours is a reasonable expectation. Some insiders suggest that if you're looking for 'bang-for-your-buck', eau de parfum is a good bet as it is generally quite a bit cheaper than the parfum. Because it can still be quite strong, apply lightly for day and more generously when you're dressing up.

Eau de toilette (aka EDT) is lighter: somewhere between 5–15 per cent of aromatic ingredients in that water/alcohol base. The name? 'Toilet water' isn't exactly romantic, so it may help to know that it came from the French phrase 'faire sa toilette': the ritual of getting dressed and ready, in which putting on perfume (in whatever strength) is the final, glamorous gesture. (Ideal for work, for interviews, for when you want to wear scent for your personal pleasure, rather than to help get you 'noticed'.) Two to three hours of wear is all you can reasonably expect before the last traces drift away. (Nevertheless, eau de toilette is the bestselling scent strength in the UK and many other countries.)

Eaux de Cologne are lighter still and often feature more will o' the wisp, 'volatile' ingredients such as citrus and herbs in the blend – a traditional hangover from the early recipes for this type of scent. But eaux de Cologne not only lack the base notes to 'tether' them: they feature between just 2–5 per cent of aromatic compounds: an airier, more dilute formula altogether. Great for a 'wake-up' splash in the morning – or a cool-down in the day – but don't expect this strength of scent to hang around for long: you'll be lucky to get

two hours out of an eau de Cologne.

Eau fraîche is another phrase you'll sometimes see on a label: a light, scented, generally summer 'refresher', occasionally formulated without any alcohol at all (and sometimes available as 'limited edition' summer versions of popular perfumes). Expect around 3 per cent concentration of perfumed oils, and a life of no more than a couple of hours.

Aftershave is roughly 1–3 per cent

concentration, although men's Colognes or even eau de parfum options are also available for some scents, mirroring the concentrations above. (Aftershaves also sometimes contain aloe or other balm-like ingredients in the formulation for skin soothing: they are designed for freshly shaven skin, give a quick euphoric 'burst' of scent and swiftly disappear.)

Very, very occasionally you'll see the phrase eau généreuse or eau d'abondance on a label – generally on a

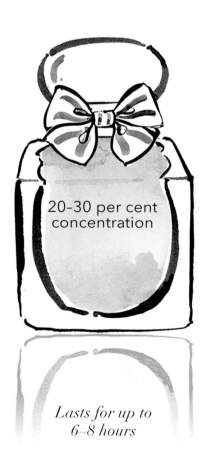

Perfume *(Parfum)*

20–30 per cent concentration

Lasts for up to 6–8 hours

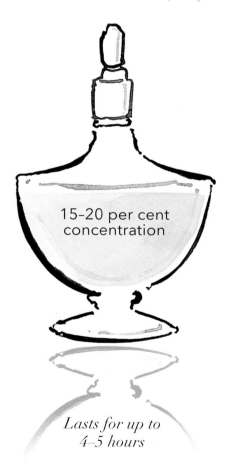

Eau de Parfum *(EDP)*

15–20 per cent concentration

Lasts for up to 4–5 hours

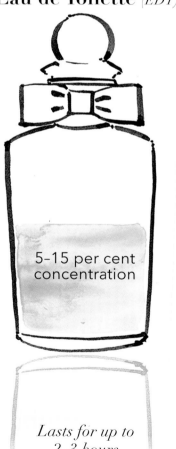

Eau de Toilette *(EDT)*

5–15 per cent concentration

Lasts for up to 2–3 hours

whacking great bottle, designed to be splashed with abandon. The phrase refers to the size of the bottle rather than the concentration: generally, these contain an eau de toilette or eau de Cologne strength.

So: above are the most common phrases and strengths. But it's not quite as straightforward as it seems because perfume houses don't only dilute their creations, depending on the strength – sometimes they do quite a bit of reformulation for each version. Which

means when you've found a fragrance you really like, do explore it in all its concentrations. You may find that you adore the eau de toilette, but the parfum's too old-fashioned or, conversely, that you're crazy for the perfume, but the eau de parfum doesn't seem to share its magic. It's another example of why there really is nothing – but nothing – like trying a fragrance on your skin before buying. Even if you have to do the perfume-spritzing equivalent of kissing a few frogs, before you find your ultimate match.

Eau de Cologne *(EDC)*

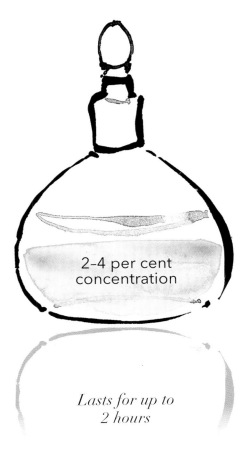

2–4 per cent concentration

Lasts for up to 2 hours

Eau Fraîche

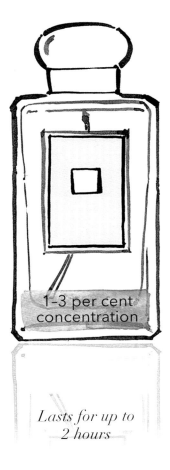

1–3 per cent concentration

Lasts for up to 2 hours

TIP

If you have dry skin, apply fragrance more often

And whatever your skin type, a technique known as layering will help make your scent last longer: if the perfume you love has a matching bath product, body lotion/cream or powder, all of these really will turbocharge the staying power of your perfume, because they give something to 'cling to'. If those bath and body treats aren't available (or are beyond your budget), a rich but unscented cream is the best 'primer' for perfume: try to avoid anything that clashes with your favourite scent. (Although anyone who's familiar with the notes and 'families' of their fragrances and what's in their body products can experiment with some interesting D-I-Y 'layering' effects – even if it would probably give the 'nose' who created your perfume an attack of the vapours). Chanel, Guerlain and L'Occitane also make specific creams for applying before fragrance, designed to complement their own portfolio of perfumes and make them last longer on the skin. (We've tried them, though, and they fare quite well with *any* fragrance you choose to apply on top, not just the creations from those brands.)

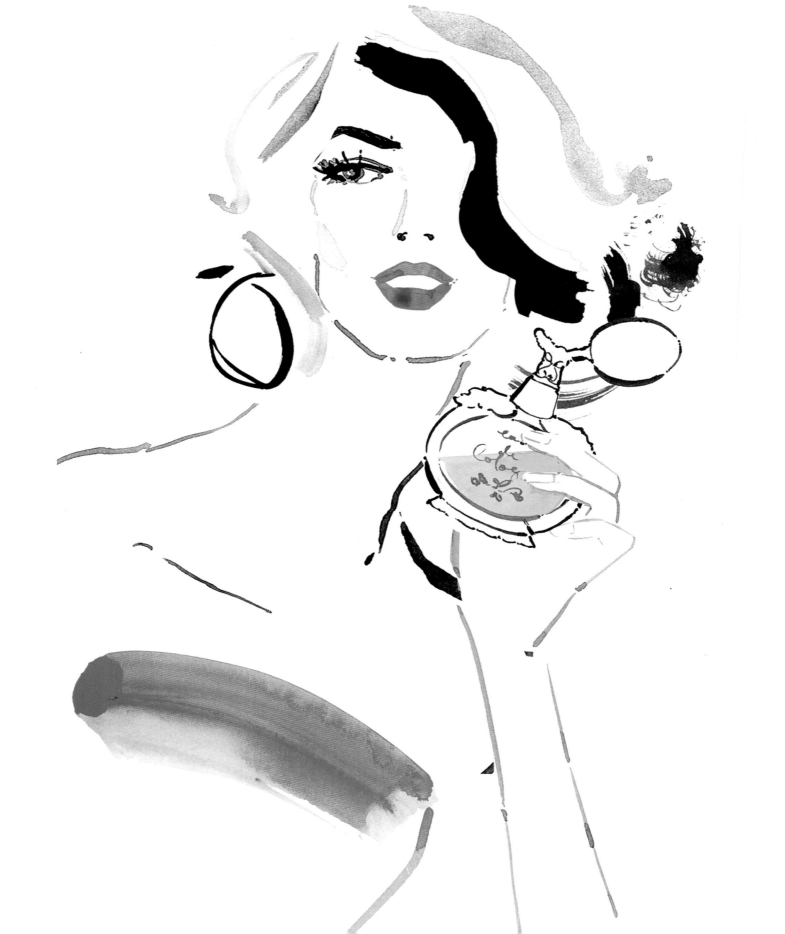

"

Smell is a potent wizard that transports us across thousands of miles and all the years you have lived

"

Helen Keller

how to find your next scent love

Fragrance isn't your groceries. It isn't your underwear (leaving out those who wear La Perla or Agent Provocateur every single day). Potentially, your perfume is something that you'll be remembered by - by friends and family - long after you've gone. (We all have those treasured memories of mothers, grandmothers and great-aunts bending down to kiss us goodnight.)

We don't believe that fragrance shopping should be rushed – not least because there is a huge amount of pleasure to be had from the quest for something new to dab or spritz. The recent explosion of interest in perfume – not just wearing it, but its creation – means that there are more (and more interesting) places to explore fragrance. We suggest you sniff them out. (On pages 158–161, we share some of our global favourites.)

But whatever your destination, the following will make it easier to find your new 'love':

There is a huge amount of pleasure to be had from the quest for something new to dab or spritz

Don't eat spicy foods or garlic the night before. These literally 'seep' through the skin and change how a fragrance smells. Fact. You may not be able to smell that curry – but it will still have an effect.

If you wear deodorant, make sure it's unscented. You don't want a clash.

Wear clean clothes. Experts recommend a clean white T-shirt is best of all for perfume shopping (though go easy on the fabric conditioner, which can also clash). Fragrance clings to clothes and influences what you're smelling, and traces of any perfumes you already wear will be detectable on cashmere jumpers, wool jackets or anything made of silk, especially.

Ideally, shop in the morning. Your nose is definitely fresher, and the department stores and perfumeries are generally emptier. If possible, do it on a day off, so you're not rushed: make a special expedition.

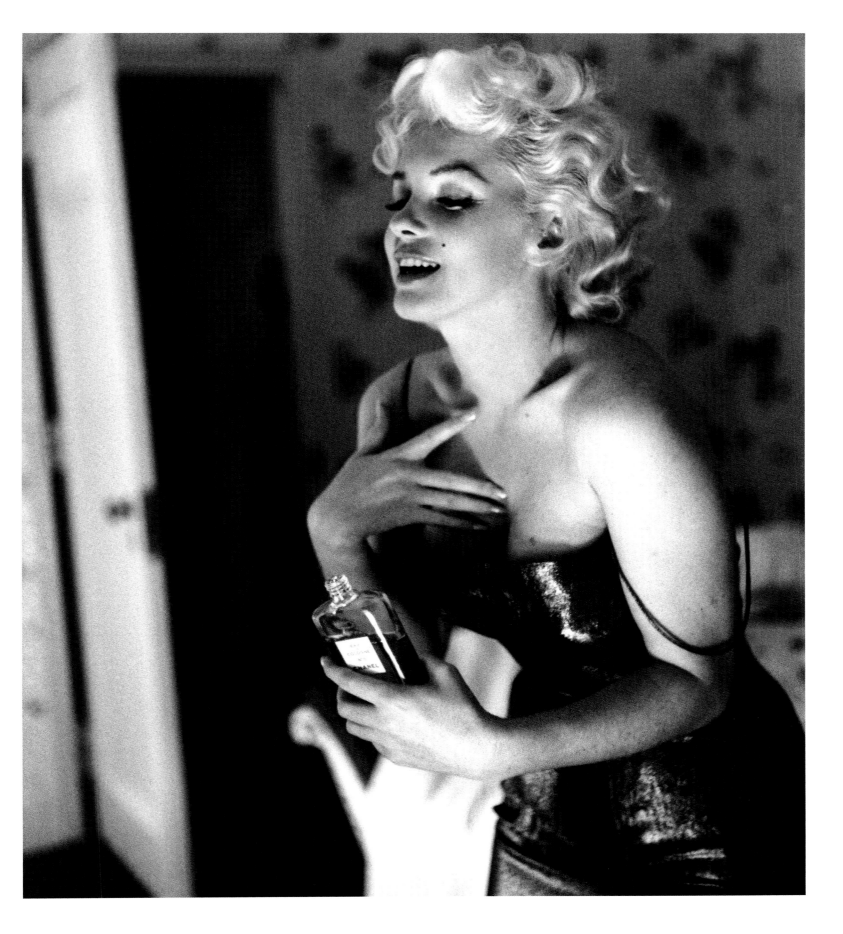

Think about dressing the way you'd actually dress to wear the type of scent you're searching for. That might mean jeans for something weekend-y, a pair of higher heels and maybe a little bit more make-up if you're on the hunt for something for night-time. If you're going to talk to a consultant for recommendations, it will help if she can clock your lifestyle.

Dodge the 'guerilla sprayers'. This is going to make us unpopular, but we generally advise giving a wide berth to the consultants who try to spray you with the 'next big thing' on your way into a store. Sure, it's fun to smell the 'scent-of-the-moment': the buzzy perfume from this celebrity or that designer, or the one you've just seen lavishly advertised on a 40ft screen in your local multiplex. But it's not guaranteed to suit you, no matter how you rather long for it to. And by the time you've got the 'latest thing' all over you (these professional sprayers tend to be ultra-generous with the spritzing), it's going to be near-impossible to smell anything else.

Ideally, carry blotters with you when you go shopping. Packs of these are generally only available via wholesalers, in massive bulk – but we offer packs of blotters to subscribers to The Perfume Society (www.perfumesociety.org), which are perfect for scent shopping. Blotters are little strips or squares of blotting-type paper, which you spray with scents before applying perfume to the skin, in order to help you narrow down the possibilities. Some counters offer their own blotters. Use them. Everyone, but everyone, gets perfume 'amnesia': it's impossible to remember what you sprayed where. And if you spray straight away on to your skin, you'll soon run out of places to try fragrances – almost certainly long before you've found something you love.

> " *This is about your feelings and memories – and if you are so unsure about whether you like the smell of something that you've got to ask someone else's opinion, it's probably not right anyway* "

Use a pen or pencil to label every blotter. Boring and laborious, yes. (And we know we sound schoolteacher-y, here.) But it is honestly and truly the only way you'll remember what you've sprayed. (Even we can't, so we've trained ourselves to write down the fragrance name before spraying.)

If you're shopping with a friend, try to be immune to their impressions. Perfume's entirely personal. What you love and what smells good on you is going to be different from what they love and what smells good on them. This is about your feelings and memories – and if you are so unsure about whether you like the smell of something that you've got to ask someone else's opinion, it's probably not right anyway. It's incredibly easy to be influenced by someone else's taste and presumptions about you and your style – so we'd recommend perfume shopping as a solitary pursuit, if you're up for it. If not, stick to your guns.

Spray, spray – and walk away. If you can possibly restrain yourself, initially just spray a few blotters (which you have labelled). Go off and have a coffee or a tea. Smell the blotters again, away from the over-fragranced setting of a perfume department, at your leisure. Give the perfumes time to develop and unfold, and for the initial rush of alcohol to evaporate. Eliminate the ones you don't like by smelling two blotters, one after another for comparison, and then putting aside the one you like least, and so on until you've no more than three left on your 'shortlist'. And if there's nothing that floats your boat…? Start over. As we've been known to say: a new perfume can become a long-term romance – and should be approached like a game of seduction.

Once you've 'approved' what's on a scent blotter, then (and only then) try it on your skin. Ideally, try one single perfume at a time on your skin: wrists and the crook of the elbow. Two is do-able: we all live busy lives. But never more than three, or you'll confuse your senses.

Keep a sheet of kids' stickers in your handbag to write on. Label which pulse point you've applied which scent to. We're not mad: honestly, this is what even the great 'noses' do.

Then walk away, and allow the fragrances to develop for at least an hour – but preferably overnight. This is where it's really easy to get over-eager, sniff madly and reach for the credit card. Don't do it! Where most of us go wrong is choosing on the basis of the first fleeting burst of a scent, or the middle notes (which unfurl after 10–15 minutes). You need to understand a fragrance's journey through its accords, so don't make snap judgments. Above all, you should wait for the base notes of a fragrance to emerge before you make up your mind whether to buy it or not – and these take at least two hours to unfurl properly. The base notes are mostly what you live with when you buy a perfume – and they need to speak to you. (Or preferably sing. Beautifully.)

If you're still in love with one of the scents after this, nip back another day and spray it all over. As our old friend Roja Dove (creator of Roja Parfums) once told us, 'It's the difference between looking at the dress on the hanger, and wearing it…'

Better still, ask for a sample, if the consultant has one. Wear it for a few days. Then, and only then – when you're truly happy – flex that credit card. (And if

Wait for the base notes of a fragrance to emerge before you make up your mind whether to buy it or not

this all sounds s-o-o-o-o-o laborious, in a world in which there's too-much-to-do-in-too-little-time? Just ask yourself: how many bottles of fragrance have you bought in the past – and fallen out of love with, almost faster than you can say eau de parfum?)

Be conscious that consultants are frequently on commission. In department stores, most consultants can only ever recommend the scents created by the company they work for; in some cases, the consultants may be promotional staff brought in simply for the purpose of hitting the (usually ambitious) sales target for a single high-profile scent. Yes, there are some fantastically knowledgeable consultants out there – and we take our hats off to their passion and knowledge, but…

Don't feel pressured into buying. Ever. End. Of.

The bottom line? As the song goes, 'You can't hurry love'. And since every new fragrance is like a new love affair, that applies to perfume shopping, too.

CAN FR.eD HELP?

There's a handful of specialist Apps and 'virtual fragrance advisors' out there that, based on what you already like, can make some educated suggestions for fragrances to try which are more likely to hit the spot than most. (Check out Givaudan's iPerfumer iPhone App, or try an online consultation at www.nose.fr, the website for a Parisian specialist perfumery, which makes mostly suggestions from the niche end of the perfume market.) We're rather proud that the first 'virtual fragrance' advisor, FR.eD – short for 'Fragrance Editor' – was created by one of this book's authors, Lorna McKay, back in 1992. Following a high-tech makeover, he currently makes an appearance on our www.perfumesociety.org website, where you can tap in fragrances you wear and let FR.eD help you take a shortcut to other perfumes you should try, out of the thousands on the market.

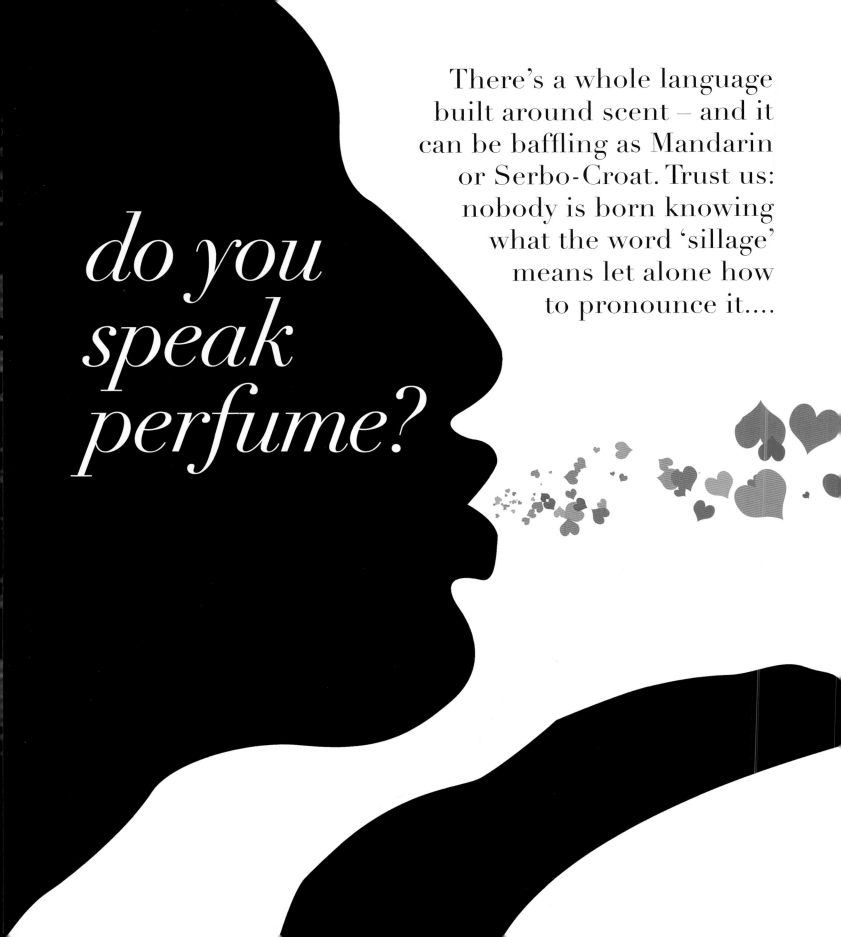

do you speak perfume?

There's a whole language built around scent – and it can be baffling as Mandarin or Serbo-Croat. Trust us: nobody is born knowing what the word 'sillage' means let alone how to pronounce it....

First of all, let's look at the 'perfume pyramid'. It's the industry standard for showing how a fragrance is composed. Lately, more 'linear' fragrances are being introduced: a form of fragrance construction that gives a more immediate sense of how the fragrance is going to smell over time – but most people follow this structure…

How fragrance is constructed

Top notes Perfumery materials evaporate at different rates because their molecules are different sizes. The smallest ones are quickest to disappear into the air, which is why citrussy Colognes don't last long on the skin; those molecules are tiny. Most fruit notes are top notes, too, really only detectable in the first minutes after application of a fragrance.

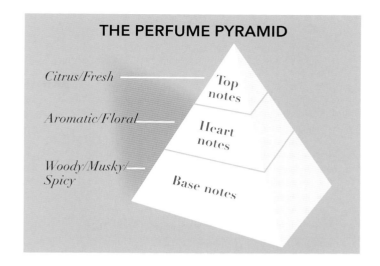

THE PERFUME PYRAMID

Citrus/Fresh ——————— Top notes

Aromatic/Floral——————— Heart notes

Woody/Musky/Spicy ——————— Base notes

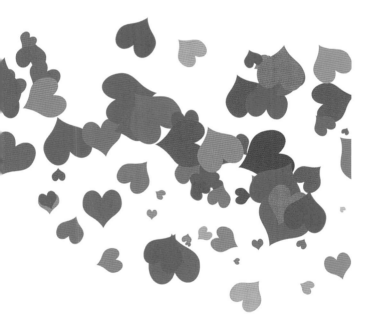

Heart notes (aka middle notes) The heart of a fragrance very often contains two 'pillars', rose and jasmine, along with other floral notes such as iris, ylang ylang, violet, etc. These are medium-sized molecules, making up the heart of a fragrance, which generally develop after 10–15 minutes and stay longer on the skin than top notes.

Base notes These larger molecules sit on the skin for hours; some also sometimes double as 'fixatives', slowing down the evaporation of top and middle notes, and so help the perfume to last longer on the skin. Base notes include many of the animalic notes – musks, civet (synthetic, nowadays), ambergris – as well as spices (cinnamon, vanilla), mosses (especially oakmoss) and woods, such as sandalwood and cedarwood. As you can read on page 29, it's essential you like the base of a fragrance, as these are the notes that you really live with once the top and heart have dissipated.

Denyse Beaulieu articulately describes the unfolding of a fragrance (in her book, *The Perfume Lover*): 'The development of a fragrance is like a relay race: when a material evaporates, another material or another 'accord' – notes that are 'played' at the same time, like a piano chord, and create a different effect when combined than individually – take up the slack to continue the story.'

Musical composers produce compositions for the ear; perfume composers produce them to delight our noses

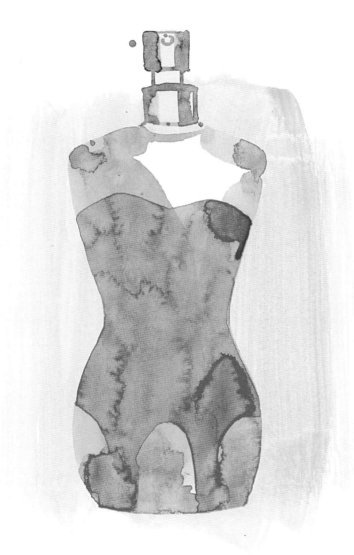

Absolute Absolutes are very precious in perfumery. They're natural fragrance materials that have been extracted from various plants – rose, jasmine, etc – usually through the use of a solvent. (Hexane is widely used.) The solution that is produced through this extraction is filtered and then concentrated through steam distillation to produce a waxy substance called a 'concrete'. The fragrant compounds are further extracted from this with alcohol (ethanol), and when that evaporates, an oil – the absolute – is left behind. It's time-consuming, expensive – and it's no wonder that the highly concentrated fragrant material left at the end is so pricy.

Accord Accords are combinations of single notes, which are used to produce other fragrant effects. An accord might be two ingredients; it could run into several hundred. Many 'noses' work on accords quite separately to their commercial perfume creations – like composers coming up with pleasing combinations of musical notes. They may later take them 'off the shelf', to create specific effects in more complex creations. The most famous accord of all in perfumery is the Guerlinade: a top-secret combination of notes, which gives a specific and unmistakable 'signature' (we'd call it warm, sweet and fuzzy) to everything the Guerlain perfume house produces.

Aldehydic Aldehydes are a family of synthetic notes (their most famous use is in Chanel No. 5). Sometimes a bit starchy, they add sparkle to the first impression of a perfume. The 'whoosh' can be a bit like unstoppering a bottle of champagne.

Animalic Animalic notes were used in perfumery for centuries (millennia, even) for their sexy qualities – even though, when smelled 'neat', most of the materials are completely horrendous, and it's mind-boggling how the early perfumers got the idea that these ingredients would smell good on humans. In small doses, however, they add depth and sensuality to perfumes. Civet (from the civet cat/weasel), musk (musk deer) and castoreum (beaver) are all animalic notes – although they've mostly been replaced by synthetics, due to conservation/cruelty concerns. Some plants can have 'animalic' qualities, too, such as cumin oil, with its warm sweatiness.

Anosmia This is the inability to smell odours. Some individuals can suffer from anosmia after a drug reaction or a knock to the head; the condition can be permanent and affect quality of life. Much more widespread, though, is an inability to make out some perfume ingredients that others can smell, most commonly, some of the synthetic musks.

Aromatic Referring to the green, bracing, 'nose-opening' qualities of herb garden ingredients such as lavender, sage and rosemary – see also camphorous.

Balsamic You've probably tasted balsamic vinegar – but what's that got to do with perfume? (Vinegar and perfume: hmmm, not an alluring link.) Balsamic generally refers to the use of resins in a perfume, but also to a fragrance impression that's sweet, soft and warm. (Not at all vinegary!) Oriental perfumes often have a balsamic quality.

Camphorous/camphoraceous Notes that have a clean, fresh, medicinal smell – bracing, basically. The adjective doesn't just refer to camphor itself (that mothball-y scent); rosemary, lavender/lavandin, pine and other conifer oils are all camphoraceous.

Chypre A family of fragrances that are an interplay of floral, citrus, mossy and ambery notes, almost always including oakmoss, labdanum (cistus), patchouli and bergamot. Although chypre-style fragrances are said to date right back to the Roman Empire and were fashionable at the time of Marie Antoinette, the modern era of chypre fragrances really began with a fragrance called, simply, Chypre, launched by François Coty in 1917. The term chypre is French for Cyprus: it was adopted because many of the fragrance ingredients in this style of perfume flourish in the Mediterranean.

Composition Every fragrance is a composition: a blend of (hopefully) harmoniously adjusted individual notes. We often find musical references useful when it comes to perfume, because the same language is used across both art forms. Musical composers produce compositions for the ear; perfume composers produce them to delight our noses.

Decant In the US, in particular, specialist websites offer 'decants', in which a larger bottle of perfume is decanted into small trial vials for sampling by customers. We're all for sampling when manufacturers have closely monitored the process to ensure that what a potential customer smells is the real thing – but there's no way of knowing how well a fragrance that has been 'decanted' has been stored, how old it is, or even whether it's the most recent version of that perfume on the market.

Dry-down The final phase of a fragrance – the 'character' that appears several hours after application. Perfumers consider this the most important phase of a perfume's development, paying great attention to the base notes and the perfume's 'tenacity' – and we agree.

Factice Pronounced 'fact-ees', this is a 'dummy' bottle, used in a shop's display or window: the contents aren't actually perfume. Very occasionally, a shop will accidentally sell a factice to a customer: if you ever open a bottle when you get it home

and it smells of absolutely nothing at all, they've probably made this mistake – so get right back there!

Fixative This is an ingredient used to extend the life of other, more volatile, compounds in a fragrance to prevent them dissipating too quickly. Some well-known base notes are also fixatives: benzoin, frankincense, musk, as well as orris root.

Flanker When a perfume's successful, perfume houses want to capitalise on that, so they'll often release variations (sometimes limited editions) on the original theme. These are generally packaged in the same bottle as the original, although it might have a different colour or finish, or be decorated in some way. If you like a particular fragrance and a 'flanker' emerges, it's always worth checking out.

Floralcy Basically, a slightly poncy (but nevertheless still quite widely used) word for floweriness.

Fougère Fougère means fern in French and this is the name for a fragrance family – mostly of men's scents – which are supposed to have a green, ferny feel. (Ironically, of course, ferns are scentless.) The family got its name from a scent from Houbigant called Fougère Royale, first launched in 1882, which blended synthetic coumarin with a classic eau de Cologne base of lavender, citrus and geranium, together with amber, oakmoss and musk. A lovely, if little-known, family; we suggest you make its acquaintance.

TIP

Don't rub...

We see it all the time: people rub their wrists together vigorously after applying a perfume, to try to 'spread' or 'warm' it. But as perfumer Francis Kurkdjian explains, rubbing it 'will heat it up and change the chemistry of the scent. It's like drinking champagne at the wrong temperature'. So be patient: waft your wrists about a bit – they'll dry soon enough – and your scent will a) smell the way it's meant to, and b) last longer on the skin.

Gourmand A gourmand is someone very fond of eating and drinking (sometimes, to excess…). But 'gourmand' now also refers to almost 'edible' fragrances, embracing good-enough-to-eat notes such as caramel, chocolate, vanilla, marshmallow, praline, etc. Thierry Mugler popularised gourmand fragrances with Angel, but many, many women's fragrances now have at least some gourmand elements.

Herbal Refers to a fragrance reminiscent of cut, usually dried herbs – lavender, rosemary, sage – or sometimes having a cut-grass quality.

Indolic Stay with us here. Some white flowers – such as jasmine, neroli, lilac, orange blossom and tuberose – have a sort of mothball-y quality: heavy, tarry, very strong and maybe slightly decayed, from a particular aroma component in the flower called indole. Some people also like to say that 'indoles' smell animalic, or even like poo – but in reality, indole has more of that mothball quality. In large quantities, indoles – either natural or synthetically manufactured – smell overwhelming. When expertly diluted by a perfumer, they can give a narcotic, radiant 'lift' to a perfume. But if someone uses the word indolic, they're probably referring to a richly exotic white floral smell.

Leathery Certain ingredients can conjure up the smell of leather (and of suede), giving a sort of 'gentleman's club' impression: animalic, sometimes smoky and dry, or masculine. When these are played up in a perfume, it's described as leathery. (Chanel's Cuir de Russie is a perfect leathery example.)

Linear There's a lot of talk these days about 'linear' perfumery – it's a sort of what-you-smell-is-what-you-get approach – and it's a trend because perfume houses don't have long to attract a customer's attention and are keen to give a full impression of the scent from first spritz, to encourage an instant purchase. Basically, in a linear perfume the top notes don't vary that much from the bottom notes, a slightly different approach to classic perfumery (with its 'pyramid') – but it doesn't translate as dull and boring: there are some wonderful linear perfumes out there.

Nose Someone who mixes fragrance ingredients to create perfumes and other scented products (even the leading 'noses' often work on washing powders and home fragrance products, unless they're exclusively working as in-house perfumers to the big fragrance houses). In France, a nose is 'le nez'; the word 'creator' is also used ('parfumeur créateur') in France. There are many people involved in the creation of perfumery who aren't trained noses: they're sometimes referred to as evaluators, or 'creative directors', and the industry's still trying to come up with a phrase for this valuable role which nevertheless stops slightly short of being an actual 'nose'.

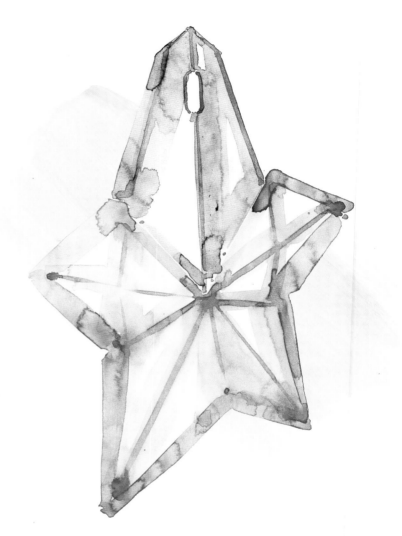

Thierry Mugler popularised gourmand fragrances with Angel, but many women's fragrances now have at least some gourmand elements

Master Perfumer The French fragrance house Firmenich awards this official title – capital 'M', capital 'P' – to a handful of perfumers who've distinguished themselves for their success and creativity within the industry. There's nothing to stop a perfumer calling himself or herself a 'master perfumer' (small 'm', small 'p') though – and it happens a lot.

Musky Almost every fragrance has a musk or two nestling somewhere in the base; there's a huge range of musks out there, which deliver different effects: white musks smell like freshly ironed linen, others are creamy and sweet and some, much more exotic. But when the term 'musky' is used to describe a perfume, it generally means it has depth and sexiness: a touch of the wild to it. (If someone tells you that you smell musky, though – and you're not wearing a musk-based perfume – you might want to do an armpit check: it can also translate as 'body odour', in human hygiene terms.)

Oriental A family of fragrances based around some of the ingredients traditionally used in Oriental and Arabic perfumery: vanilla, musk, patchouli, balsams, sandalwood, spices, etc. The character of an Oriental can be exotic, spicy, sexy – not generally for day-wear, we find.

Ozonic Think of the air right after a thunderstorm or the tang when you walk along a beach with waves crashing on the shore. An ozonic effect is created via synthetic ingredients to conjure up the smell of fresh air.

Powdery Some ingredients can give a soft, almost fuzzy quality to a perfume, almost as if it had a texture. Iris, violet, almond, heliotrope and some musks give this haziness. The effect can be more Johnson's Baby Powder, or 'Mummy's face powder', explored in an old-fashioned or a contemporary way. (Chanel No. 19 Poudré is a modern 'powdery' scent, while Guerlain Shalimar is a masterpiece of old-style powderiness.)

Rich Opulent, extravagant, intense, maybe OTT: a 'rich' fragrance isn't subtle any more than a red Ferrari is understated. Generally, rich fragrances feature lavish quantities of florals, musks or spices. We think you'll know one when you smell it.

Sillage A French word – say it 'see-ah-j' – it means 'trail' or 'wake'. It's come to mean the scent left by a person as they pass by.

Soapy Generally, soapy is a put-down – it suggests a fragrance smells like a cheap soap (rather than the glorious and generally pricier soaps out there). In reality, some 'soapy' scents can be beautiful: aldehydes can give a soapiness, as can some musks and orange blossom. If you like something, that should be good enough for you; ignore everyone else.

Soliflore A fragrance that is created to represent a single flower – lily of the valley, rose, lavender, gardenia. In reality, most 'soliflores' use many different ingredients to conjure up an apparently simple flower or plant.

Spill A 'spill' is a blotter used for trying out fragrances, made of a special absorbent type of blotting paper.

Vanillic We all know what vanilla smells like, but other ingredients – benzoin, tolu balsam, etc – can also give a vanilla-y smell. In perfume-speak, though, professionals don't say 'vanilla-y' – they say 'vanillic'.

White floral White flowers include jasmine, orange blossom, lilac, gardenia, jasmine, frangipani, tiaré, tuberose, lily of the valley, etc, all of which can have a quite hypnotic effect. A 'white floral bouquet' brings together several of these narcotic flowers in one fragrance, to ultra-feminine effect. (Because of their traditional 'white' association, white florals are often suggested as bridal perfumes.)

Woody means, well…woody! The adjective is used to describe fragrances in which the woody notes – rosewood, cedarwood, sandalwood – are played up. (Patchouli also smells 'woody', even though it's a green, leafy plant.) Masculine fragrances are more likely to be 'woody' than those specifically targeted at women.

Zesty Fresh, uplifting, invigorating, zesty fragrances capture the 'zestiness' of the oils released when you plunge your fingers into a lemon, an orange or a grapefruit to peel it.

TIP

If you want fragrance for a Christmas gift, be specific

Don't leave it to luck or chance: you'll almost certainly be disappointed. Don't even rely on heavy hints: make it clear what you want! (We leave Post-it notes with 'Dear Santa' written on them. Saves a lot of heartache, embarrassment and expense.)

signature scent 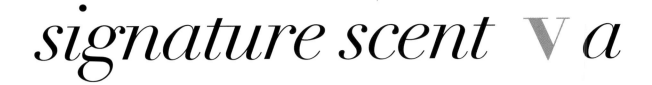 *va*

There's something wonderful about the notion that, in years to come, your children or godchildren might smell a scent on a stranger and instantly think of you. In the past, women certainly tended to have a 'signature scent', which clung to their skin and their clothes and was almost a part of their very personality. But we use the 'shoes analogy'…

Our mothers, for instance, definitely wore signature scents (Rochas Femme for Jo's mother, Estée Lauder Knowing for Lorna's) – but also had just a handful of pairs of shoes. Today, our wardrobes are way bigger, our lives infinitely more complex and busier – and a woman can be called upon to play many different roles, from CEO to mother, carer to sister, lover to PA, in the course of a single day. So will a single fragrance carry us through all those roles?

If we choose it to, of course it can. We can't tell you whether or not you're a one-scent woman, but we can tell you that if you vow you're going to be unswervingly faithful to one particular scent forever, you're missing out on a lot of intriguing dalliances: the perfume world is filled with ever-more-intriguing fragrances, and in terms of sheer sensory excitement it is worth

wardrobe of fragrances

exploring what else is out there – even if it doesn't end up on your own dressing table.

But back to the shoes analogy: would you wear a pair of tennis shoes to a ball? Or, conversely, would you really want to teeter round a farmer's market in a pair of five-inch heels? Would you wear Havaianas in winter, or snow boots in July? We think there's a lot to be said for switching perfumes not just for different times of day and night, but for mood, season and the 'role' you're about to play. (For us, applying perfume is part of getting dressed, giving a little power-boost before a business meeting, or shifting us from end-of-the-day grouchiness into a decidedly more smoochy mood for dinner à deux with our respective partners.) And the trouble with owning one scent that you wear day in, night out – as perfume expert and industry analyst Marian Bendeth observes – 'is it reveals only one dimension of our personality'. So…

Identify the 'gaps' in your fragrance wardrobe. This is the perfume equivalent of throwing open your closet at the beginning of the season and deciding: I'm short of T-shirts, I could do with a smart summer frock, or what I really need is a pair of dressy heels to take me from desk to dinner. Have you got the basics covered: something for day, something for night (could be a stronger version of the same scent), something for summer, something for winter? We find that some fragrances are almost

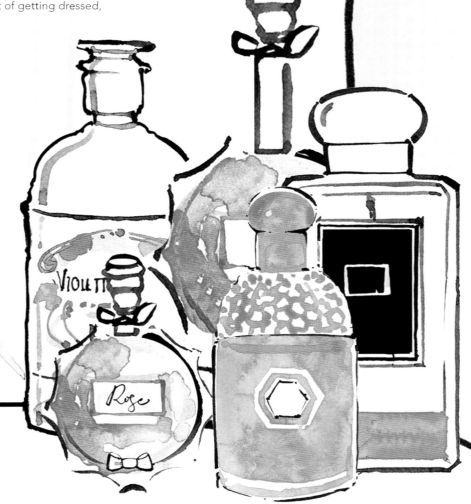

impossible to wear 'out of season': Jo, for instance, has had a long love affair with Guerlain Mitsouko – but gets it out of her cupboard at exactly the same time as her winter opaque tights. If you don't know where to start, a fragrance consultant in a specialist perfumery or a department store should be able at least to help point you in the direction of choices more appropriate for different times of day or season.

Be aware that hot weather affects fragrance. Another good reason to have something lighter and airier for summer: heat not only limits the lifespan of some ingredients on the skin, but intensifies others: heavy, musky, woody scents can become overpowering in the heat. According to our perfume creator friend Azzi Glasser, 'Fresh marine, green, herbal and citrus accords all work well in summer, as they represent freshness, energy and, in some cases, coolness.'

Go for something sensual for night. You probably want something slightly stronger (an eau de parfum or even parfum/perfume), which makes more of an impact – and maybe has more of a sexy, 'smouldering' base.

Travel a richer path for autumn/winter. There's nothing to say you can't wear a classic Cologne all year round, but we find that woodier, spicier, fruitier scents really come into their own as autumn segues into winter – and, in particular, notes such as vanilla, tonka, incense, musks, creamy woods (like sandalwood), cinnamon, nutmeg… They're sort of the olfactory equivalent of snuggling in front of a log fire beneath a cashmere blanket.

And try a 'calm-down' fragrance, for your desk. With lavender being one of the few aromatherapy oils scientifically proven to have a calming effect, it can be worth having a spray based on genuine lavender essential oil within reach to prevent at-desk meltdowns (and in a world in which there's too-much-to-do-in-too-little-time, we all have them). This doesn't have to be an actual perfume: just something you spray into the air around you. (If it's alcohol-based, without too many oils, it may also work as a computer screen cleaner on an e-cloth, doing triple duty by freshening the surrounding air while it soothes your neurotransmitters.)

Play with perfumes on holiday. We never go anywhere without smelling what's on offer locally – either small in boutiques, or souks, or large department stores (although all too often, the offerings in those are pretty global, rather than destination-specific). The advantage of shopping for a new scent while you're away is that you're likely to be less rushed and may notice things you wouldn't during normal, probably stressed, day-to-day life. We absolutely love buying a new perfume on our travels, wearing it in a particular city or holiday destination – and knowing that

My grandmother Estée Lauder always said you wouldn't wear the same dress to play tennis and go out to dinner, so why would you wear the same fragrance?

Aerin Lauder

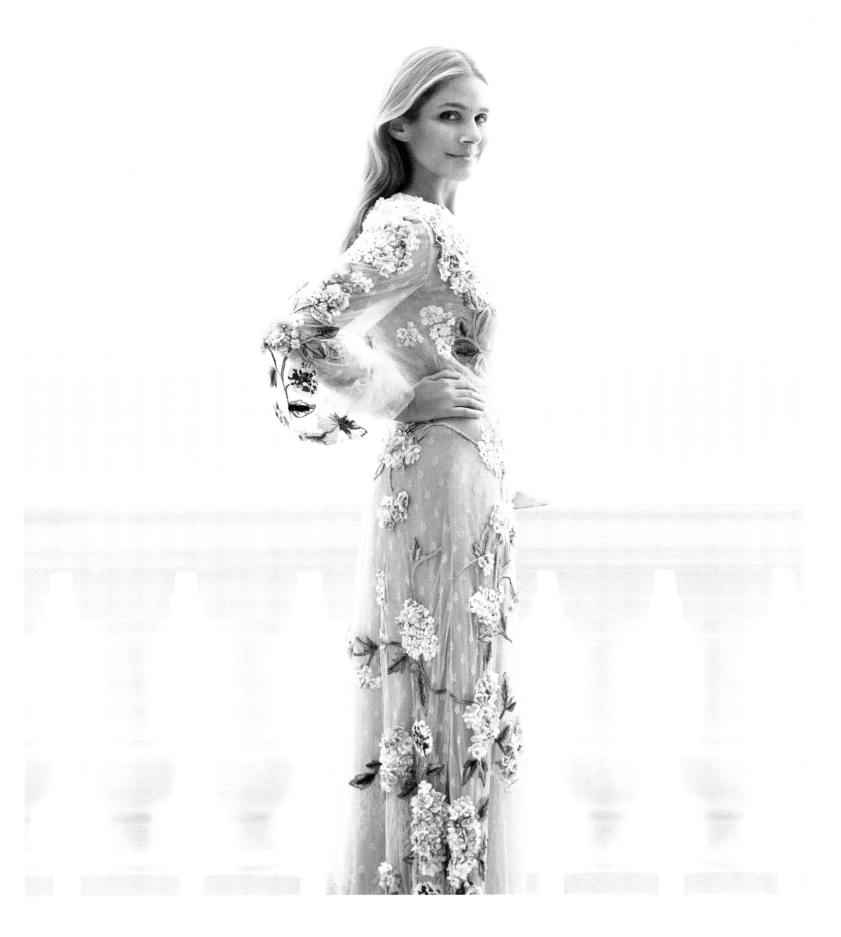

Each great new discovery reminds me that perfume is a simple pleasure, but it can be a potent accessory. It cheers me up when I feel down. It makes me feel elegant, focused, playful, powerful. It helps me indulge my fantasies and my wanderlust. How could I wear only one…?

**Victoria Frolova, Bois de Jasmin
perfume blogger**

when we're back home again, it will transport us back to that place in a millisecond. (Always being conscious of the advice above, though, that perfumes don't necessarily behave the same in different climates.)

Be on a permanent fragrance 'treasure hunt'. Sometimes you want to make a 'mission' out of shopping for perfume – see pages 26–29 – but, at the same time, never miss out on the opportunity just to sniff around and smell what's out there. Any time you're in a boutique, at a Duty Free counter (or on your global travels), have a sniff of the bottles that your eye's attracted to. (That's not quite as shallow as it sounds: as you can read on pages 80–81, fragrance houses invest a huge amount in trying to ensure the bottle perfectly represents the mood of the scent inside.) Spray some blotters (always labelling them first – see page 28) – and smell them later.

And if you do just want to 'find your signature'? To be honest, most women (and men) we know have a go-to perfume that triggers an immediate sensory response whenever we spray it, bringing back a memory of a particular place or person. Everyone should try to find a scent that makes you feel like a knockout version of yourself, something to turn to when you feel down, or you don't have a lot of time to think about what to put on. Whether you stick to this fail-safe option 24/7, 365 days a year, or turn to it more occasionally to nudge you into a better, perhaps more sociable mood, is entirely up to you.

Your wardrobe can be as small and streamlined as you like – or as varied as your budget (and the space on your dressing table) permits. The one piece of advice we would add, though, is that when choosing any fragrance, follow your own instincts – and your nose – rather than the clever and often extravagant marketing of the fragrance industry.

We think there's another very good reason to switch between two or more scents. The nose very rapidly becomes accustomed to a particular fragrance and barely registers it any more. We find that swapping and switching keeps our nose 'on its toes', and we notice our perfume more when it's not just 'part of the furniture', or mere wallpaper to our lives.

And when you're looking for something sexy…

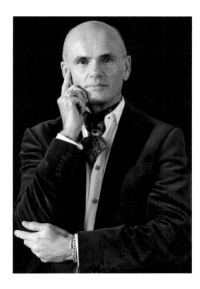

Since the dawn of time, scent has attracted us to other human beings – and them to us. Today, the reason many of us wear fragrance is to seduce. Not always – but sometimes. (Even if we don't admit it to ourselves.) So if you want a come-hither scent, you might want to modify your tactics. We asked Roja Dove, the perfume expert who now has his own signature Roja Parfums line, to advise on shopping for a specifically seductive fragrance, because this requires a slightly different approach…

● 'It's no good shopping for a seductive scent when you're in "work mode". If you dress more like a femme fatale, the fragrance consultants will see you differently – and suggest sexier scents. Maybe try fragrance shopping one evening, setting aside an hour before a date or special event.'

● 'The most seductive fragrances are base-note-heavy, featuring lots of vanilla, animal notes such as musk, incense and woods like sandalwood. You'll find many of the most seductive scents in the "Oriental" family. You don't need to be an expert on this; just ask a consultant.' (In all other respects, follow the general advice we've just shared with you.)

● And once you've bought your sexy scent? 'To turbocharge a fragrance's seductive power, don't put it behind your ears,' says Roja. 'The spot above the collarbone is better – he'll smell it when he whispers in your ear – and around the navel is a hotspot, too. Remember, scent rises – so try a dab behind knees and ankles.'

TIP *Give a perfume you're considering a 'workout'…*

We like this, from perfume blogger The Non-Blonde (see page 164 for more about her). 'It's not very likely that you'll get to test a perfume in several extreme weather conditions. But you do want to know how you're going to smell when the heat is on and the sweat is pouring. I'm not telling you to go and fumigate your fellow gym-goers with Angel, but try to do a quick workout at home, go for a brisk walk or just carry your laundry up and down the stairs enough times to work up a sweat. Does the perfume still work?'

how the *magic* *of* scent *works on* the mind

We love the quote from the deaf and blind American author and lecturer Helen Keller, about scent: 'Smell is a potent wizard that transports you across thousands of miles and all the years you have lived.' But just why does fragrance have the power to whisk us through time and space? The whole psychology of scent is quite fascinating

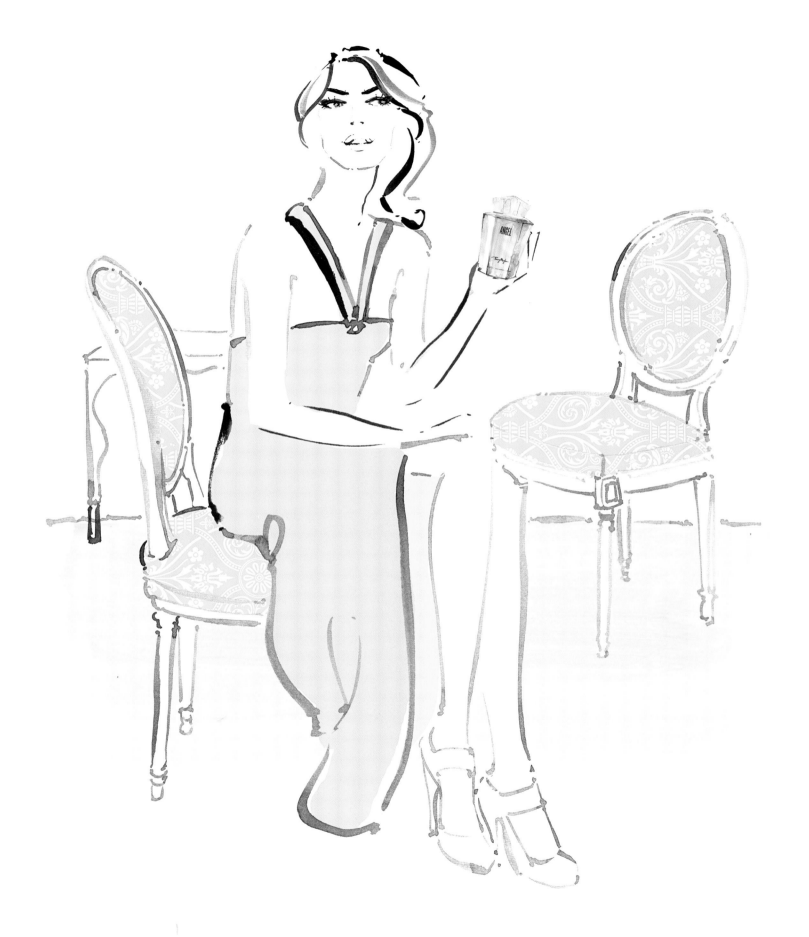

One sniff and you're somewhere else. In your granny's greenhouse. At summer camp. In the corridors of school. A whiff of something can be so evocative that it truly can be like time-travelling. But why, oh why, is smell so intimately linked with memory in this way? One reason is that the olfactory receptors are directly connected to the limbic system, the most ancient and primitive part of the brain, which is thought to be the seat of emotion, and for storing all our emotional memories.

And so a smell can very soon become associated with a particular person, a moment in time or a place. It happens so fast that by the time we correctly label a smell as – for instance – lemon or vanilla, it's already activated the limbic system and triggered a deep-seated emotional response. Sometimes, we may not even know why we have an intense reaction to a smell – intense love, intense disgust. Amazingly, that may have started before we were born: research suggests that some smell preferences may even develop in the womb.

No two individuals' smell preferences are ever going to be the same. It's intensely personal, which is why we're against

TIP

Remember: the more you smell, the more you learn

If you live or work near a perfume store or department store, take a little detour through the fragrance department each time you visit, and take away one or two scented (and labelled) blotters. Go online and do a little bit of research about the perfumes: the notes, the families, the story. It's a weird but physiological fact: just like wine, the more you know, the more enjoyment you'll get out of the whole universe of smell.

A whiff of something can be so evocative that it truly can be like time-travelling

Although smoking doesn't always affect scores in scientific smell tests, it's widely believed to reduce sensitivity to aromas, according to The Social Issues Research Centre's The Smell Report.

perfume 'snobbery'. How can it be 'right' or 'wrong' to like particular smells, when that may be shaped by something that happened before we were born? Or some other life event. Jo, for instance, once got very sick in Africa and lay feverishly in a bed near a window with the scent of jasmine wafting through it on a sea breeze. For years afterwards – two decades, almost – one of the perfume world's most exquisite ingredients made her feel nauseous.

That's not 'wrong'. That's not 'right'. If you love the smell of roads being tarred, or felt-tip pens, or mothballs, we don't think that's weird at all. (Compare and contrast with Ethiopia, where the Daasanach tribe smear cow manure on their bodies, because the smell of the cattle signals fertility and high status.) In one study, responses to the question 'What are your favourite smells?' included lots generally regarded as unpleasant (think: petrol and even body perspiration!), while some scents usually viewed as pleasant – such as flowers (as with Jo's own experience, above) – were violently disliked by some of those individuals surveyed.

What the nose knows

Compared to the sense of smell of a wild animal (and plenty of domestic ones, come to that), ours is a six-stone weakling. But it's still pretty acute: we're able to detect smells in infinitesimal quantities, and can recognise thousands of different smells. (And it's always possible to do even better, as The Perfume Society's 'Improve Your Sense of Smell' workshops set out to do; see www.perfumesociety.org for details.)

There are two patches, high up in the nose, which are made up of 'olfactory receptors'. We have five or six million of these (yellowish) cells, apparently – compared to a rabbit's 100 million, and 220 million in a dog. (Which clearly explains why dogs are deployed as drug sniffers, by the police and in airports, rather than humans!) Yet through these sensitive receptors, we are nevertheless able to detect some substances at the incredibly low concentration of less than one part in several billion parts of air.

Smell, of course, is inextricably linked to the sense of taste. Those who've lost their sense of smell often report that food has lost almost all flavour, too. Just the simplest exercise will demonstrate how crucial our noses are to what our palates detect. Hold your nose and put a square of chocolate in your mouth (Green & Black's is obviously preferable!). Savour it for 30 seconds, allowing it to melt and chewing it lightly. Then, and only then, release your nose – and you'll experience a 'taste explosion'. The so-called 'taste buds' on our tongues can only distinguish five qualities: sweet, sour, bitter, salt and 'umami', a Japanese word for 'savouriness'. (Although in Ayurvedic cookery, they recognise two extra qualities: pungent and astringent, which we certainly identify with.) All other 'tastes' are detected by the olfactory receptors high up in the nasal passages.

By the age of eight, our sense of smell has generally reached its full power. Women, meanwhile, generally seem to have a more accurate and acute sense of smell: women consistently out-perform men in tests of smelling ability. (Try this at home, we dare you!)

How well you 'hang on to' your ability to smell, meanwhile, may well depend on your overall general health. Some smell researchers suggest that this aromatic 'acuity' can decline from our twenties onwards (one scary experiment even indicated this can start at the age of 15). But other scientists have noted that a lot of it is down to overall health and well-being: some healthy 80-year-olds have the same olfactory 'prowess' as young adults. The bottom line: look after yourself, and you're looking after your sense of smell.

And one word of advice: we recommend avoiding nasal sprays. A fascinating and deeply chilling book, *Remembering Smell: A Memoir of Losing – and Discovering – the Primal Sense* by Bonnie Blodgett, is one woman's personal account of what happened after the injudicious use of a cold remedy, squirted up her nose, which first gave her 'phantosmia' – a period of smelling heinous phantom burning-rubber-like smells – and then settle into 'anosmia', or total, nightmarish loss of her sense of smell...It's a great read.

> *By the age of eight, our sense of smell has generally reached its full power*

TIP *Apply perfume before jewellery, always*

Spraying perfume on to porous jewellery such as pearls or resin can damage the surface, while in some cases perfume can interact with metals - watch bands, etc - to alter the character of the scent. (Gold is fine, though - as are diamonds!)

scents of time

Ever since man (and probably woman) first burned aromatic ingredients – as an offering to the gods, as well as (we imagine) for personal enjoyment – perfume's history has been inextricably linked with our own. We could write an entire book about fragrance and history (maybe one day we will!), but meanwhile, here are some landmarks in scented time...

4500BC The very first use of fragrance that we know of, in China, where aromatic products and a description of their uses was recorded.

3500BC Egyptian tomb writings reveal that Ancient Mesopotamians and Egyptians burned incense – which it was believed connected humans with the gods. Egyptians also lit incense in the home to create harmony between body and soul. And archaeologists have even

now uncovered a Perfume Room at Edfu, a particularly well-preserved Egyptian temple.

Perfume was central to life in Ancient Greece, too. The art of perfume-making is thought to have begun in Crete, where they experimented with extraction techniques incorporating boiled herbs and flowers, and infusing the extracted scents in oils. At one point, perfume was so popular that the politician Solon

The dawn of perfume...

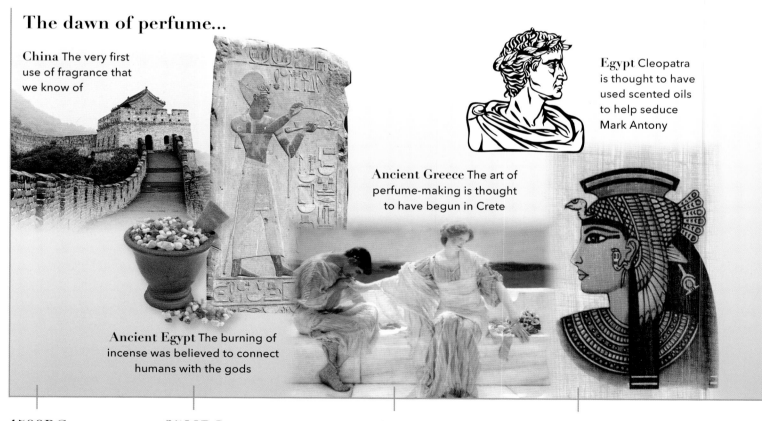

China The very first use of fragrance that we know of

Ancient Egypt The burning of incense was believed to connect humans with the gods

Ancient Greece The art of perfume-making is thought to have begun in Crete

Egypt Cleopatra is thought to have used scented oils to help seduce Mark Antony

| 4500BC | 3500BC | 700BC | 41BC |

allegedly banned it temporarily, to prevent an economic crisis. It was worn by men and women, was central to worship – used for pleasing the gods – and was integral to cleanliness, too.

41BC Cleopatra, Queen of Egypt, so loved aromatics that she had the sails of her boat coated with scented oils before setting out to sea. And she is thought to have used scented oils to help seduce Mark Antony, the Roman Consul who became her lover.

Under the influence of the Middle East and Greece, the Romans fell in love with perfume. Initially, perfume was only used for religious events and important funerals, but at Rome's official 'orgy', the Bacchanalia, Emperor Nero sprayed dinner guests with rose water perfume between courses. During the reign of

Julius Caesar, bottles of perfume were thrown to the crowds celebrating Rome's triumphs. And by the 1st century AD, Rome used about 2,800 tons of frankincense and 550 tons of myrrh a year, while the fountains of Rome flowed with rose water…

After the fall of that city, fragrance fell from grace, too. In the Middle Ages, there wasn't much of what we'd consider perfume; people simply used spices and flowers and what grew around them to make what was a distasteful-smelling world more acceptable. (When you bring your animals in to sleep indoors overnight, and there's no plumbing – well, just imagine…) Towards the end of the Middle Ages, the use of pomanders became popular, created by softening waxes and mixing them with clay and aromatic materials. They were worn about

the body (often hung around the neck, or simply carried), or used to protect clothes from insect damage in storage.

In the Arab world, the traditions of perfumery endured – and flourished. A love of fragrance has never gone out of fashion in the Arab lands. Arabia was the only place producing myrrh, cassia and labdanum, and frankincense – so valued that it could be traded for the world's costliest items. On the Silk Route, Arab merchants packed this resin on camel convoys to cross the desert, navigated by stars, trading their perfumed cargo for pearls, silks, horses, porcelain and gold.

By the 8th century, the burning of incense began to be part of religious ceremony again. In Roman Catholic and Anglican 'high church' ceremonies, incense is still burned – most of it

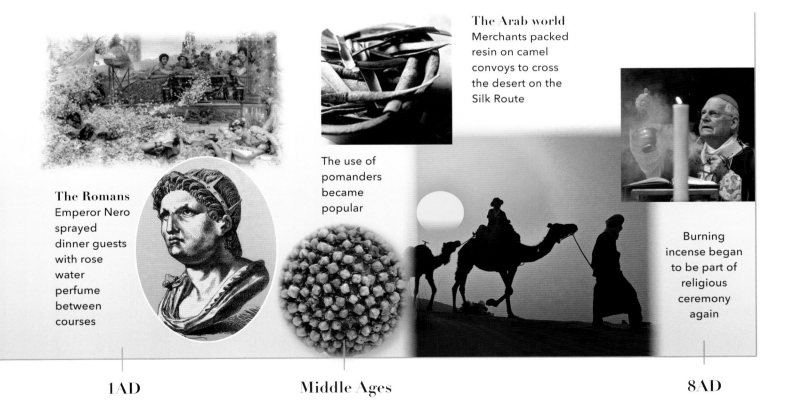

The Arab world
Merchants packed resin on camel convoys to cross the desert on the Silk Route

The Romans
Emperor Nero sprayed dinner guests with rose water perfume between courses

The use of pomanders became popular

Burning incense began to be part of religious ceremony again

1AD

Middle Ages

8AD

incorporating frankincense, which is still mainly harvested in Arabia.

The return of the Crusaders gave the use of perfume a new impetus. Victorious warriors brought home exciting perfumes for their womenfolk, from places such as Cyprus – so rich in fragrant flowers and aromatics – that had been conquered by Richard I. The recipe for rose water is thought to have been carried back by the Crusaders; it soon became a custom in the homes of the nobility to offer it to guests for rinsing hands at table. (Clearly a blessing, since the fork hadn't yet been introduced…)

It was the Italians, though, who took the art of perfumery to a new level. With Venice being such an important centre for trade, the city became the main route through which the raw materials for perfumes and incense reached Europe. For a few hundred years, then Venice

played a key role in the fragrance industry. And at the same time, clever techniques of distillation were invented, as European scientists became fascinated by the process of separating the 'essential' parts of an ingredient for use in perfume-making and medicines.

In 1370 the first alcohol-based perfume was created for Queen Elizabeth of Hungary. This toilet water was known as 'Hungary water', and included rosemary, among other aromatics. During the Renaissance, perfumes were mostly used for disguising the natural scent of leather – in gloves, handbags, leather jackets, etc – as a result of the tanning process. Meanwhile, Grasse, in France, became Europe's heartland for cultivating fragrance ingredients – and the epicentre of perfumery itself moved from Italy to France, under the influence of Queen Catherine de Medici, an Italian who married King Henry II in 1533.

It was then that the 'Maitres-Gantiers' – master glove-makers – began to dominate the fragrance industry.

Louis XIV – 'the sweetest-smelling king of all' – set off a fragrant frenzy. Louis hated baths – he's said only to have had three in his lifetime – but loved fragrance, commissioning a new scent for every day of the week. The aristocracy spent small – sometimes large – fortunes on fragrance, commissioning personal scents. Marie Antoinette was one of the most extravagant, with a personal perfumer – Jean-Louis Fargeon – while another famous beauty, Madame Tallien, liked to wash herself with perfumed milk.

But with the French Revolution, the perfume industry went into decline. Quite simply, many of its high-spending clients had lost everything – that's if they were lucky enough to escape with their heads, at a time when so many noblemen

Perfume Crusaders and the Renaissance...

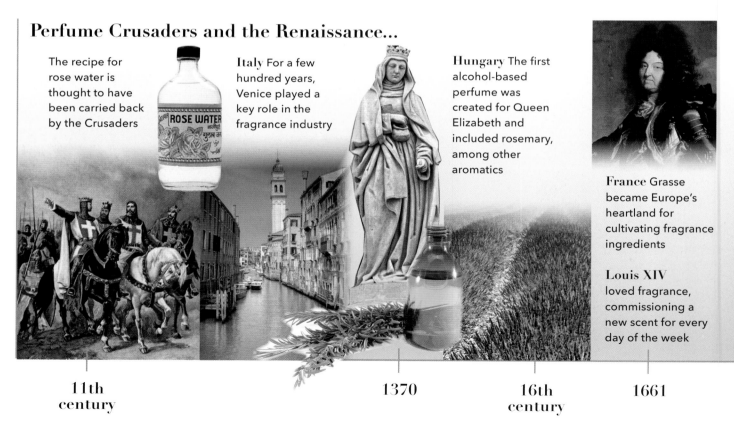

The recipe for rose water is thought to have been carried back by the Crusaders

Italy For a few hundred years, Venice played a key role in the fragrance industry

Hungary The first alcohol-based perfume was created for Queen Elizabeth and included rosemary, among other aromatics

France Grasse became Europe's heartland for cultivating fragrance ingredients

Louis XIV loved fragrance, commissioning a new scent for every day of the week

ROSE WATER

11th century   **1370**   **16th century**   **1661**

and women went to the guillotine. Napoleon and Josephine remained extravagant customers, though, throughout the Empire that followed: Napoleon had a standing order with his perfumer to deliver 50 bottles of eau de Cologne a month, while Josephine loved mignonette, hyacinths, rose, musk fragrances – and violets. (Famously, though, Napoleon liked his wife 'au naturel', once commanding her: 'Don't wash', when returning from battle.)

The Victorians were prim and proper when it came to perfume. Gentle 'single note' scents – heliotrope, lilac, rose and violets – were all that 'nice' ladies were supposed to smell of; musks and animalic notes were for 'fallen' women and prostitutes. But the Victorian era was a time of huge breakthroughs in perfume technology, with discoveries by scientists all over Europe of ways to extract – or even create synthetically –

new and exciting ingredients: vanillin, heliotropin, artificial musks, synthetic jasmine and rose.

The end of the 19th century saw the first fragrances launched that blended these synthetics with naturals. Paul Parquet created Fougère Royale for Houbigant – big on a synthetic called coumarin – while Aimé Guerlain, of the legendary Guerlain perfume house, poured generous quantities of vanillin into Jicky – forerunner of the sensual, sometimes smouldering scents to come.

François Coty introduced perfume to the 'masses', in the **early 20th century**. A savvy marketeer, this Corsican-born perfumer not only worked with exquisite bottle manufacturers like Lalique and Baccarat, but also sold plainer, smaller bottles to less wealthy customers. Coty was also the first man to allow women to sample perfumes before buying them…

The very first 'designer' fragrance was created by Paul Poiret. The creator of sensual, fluid clothes offered equally sensual fragrances to women with names such as Nuit de Chine and L'Étrange Fleur, blending synthetic and natural materials to evoke the allure and exoticism of the Orient.

In 1921, a 'mistake' led to the creation of the most famous fragrance in history. Word is that perfumer Ernest Beaux – or his lab assistant – slipped with the vial of a synthetic 'aldehyde' ingredient, adding ten times as much as the recipe specified to a sample of fragrance (one of several he was showing to designer and businesswoman Gabrielle 'Coco' Chanel). She picked out that sample from those she was shown by Beaux – No. 5, it was numbered. This sparkling floral fragrance, of course, has gone on to become the best-known fragrance of all time.

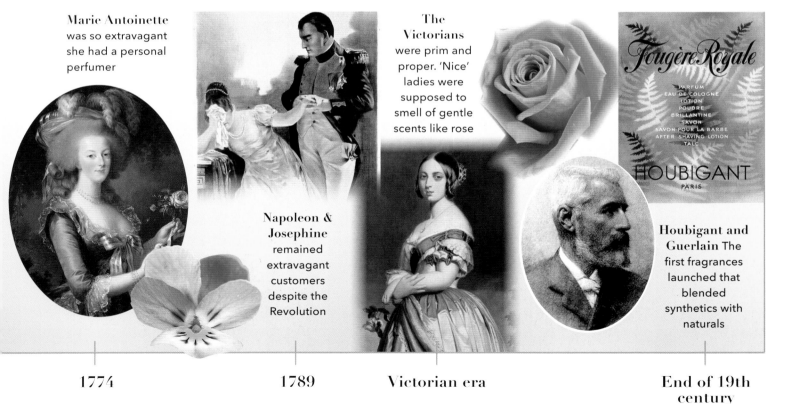

Marie Antoinette was so extravagant she had a personal perfumer

Napoleon & Josephine remained extravagant customers despite the Revolution

The Victorians were prim and proper. 'Nice' ladies were supposed to smell of gentle scents like rose

Fougère Royale
PARFUM
EAU DE COLOGNE
LOTION
POUDRE
BRILLANTINE
SAVON
SAVON POUR LA BARBE
AFTER SHAVING LOTION
TALC
HOUBIGANT
PARIS

Houbigant and Guerlain The first fragrances launched that blended synthetics with naturals

1774   1789   Victorian era   End of 19th century

The designers' domination grew – and grew. Guerlain was one of the few leading names in perfumery not linked to fashion – which hasn't held back its success, with extraordinary, enduring classics such as Mitsouko, Shalimar, Vol de Nuit and Jicky remaining in its perfume portfolio, alongside countless contemporary successes. But many of the best-known launches came from couturiers, who became as famous for the fragrant indulgences women dabbed onto their pulse points as for the clothes women draped on their bodies. Jean Patou, Elsa Schiaparelli, Lanvin and Carven all became known for stunning fragrances. It was Carven, though, who first thought up a 'launch activity' (or call it a PR stunt, if you like) for a scent: she dropped tiny green-and-white parachutes carrying samples of her debut signature scent over the skies of Paris, bringing traffic to a standstill.

In 1947, Christian Dior launched Miss Dior. Just as his New Look changed the way women wanted to dress, Dior's fragrances were hugely influential in the perfume world, with Diorissimo, Diorella and Diorama appearing on dressing tables all over the world. Truly, these were the glory days of French perfumery.

But the Americans were coming. And it was a New York businesswoman and beauty dynamo, Estée Lauder, who encouraged women to wear perfume every day, not just for special occasions. The rich, intense Oriental Youth Dew was first marketed as a bath oil – which Estée Lauder knew that women wouldn't feel guilty buying for themselves. (Before that, fragrance tended to be a gift from a loved one.)

Perfume became a daily indulgence – with more 'affordable' brands appearing on the shelves. Names such as Yardley, Lenthéric, Bourjois and Goya may not have had the cachet of the couture houses, but they could be worn and enjoyed without breaking the bank. By the 1960s, we were beginning to travel, too, and people who'd never set foot abroad could spend time browsing in foreign perfumeries and Duty Free.

In the 1970s, perfume marketing began to express women's new-found liberation. Women were starting to wear fragrance for themselves, as a form of self-expression – as well as to seduce. So we had Charlie, advertised with a woman striding out in trousers, and daring advertising campaigns that reached a climax with YSL's Opium perfume – evoking drugged intoxication, with a come-hither Jerry Hall sprawled across the pages of almost every glossy magazine you cared to open…

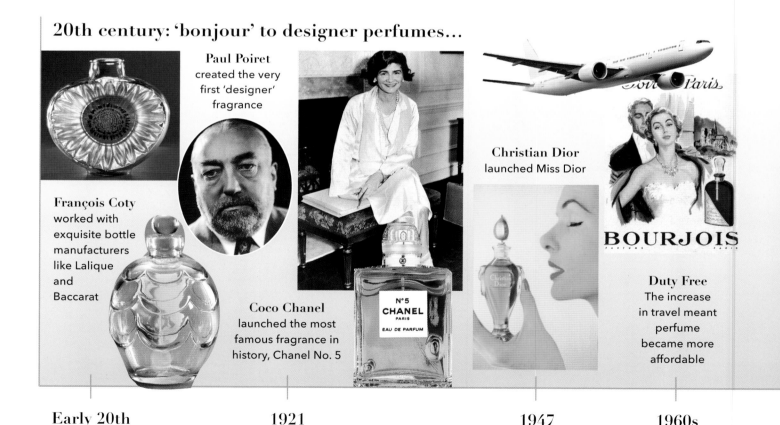

20th century: 'bonjour' to designer perfumes…

Paul Poiret created the very first 'designer' fragrance

François Coty worked with exquisite bottle manufacturers like Lalique and Baccarat

Coco Chanel launched the most famous fragrance in history, Chanel No. 5

Christian Dior launched Miss Dior

N°5 CHANEL PARIS EAU DE PARFUM

BOURJOIS

Duty Free The increase in travel meant perfume became more affordable

Early 20th century   1921   1947   1960s

The 1980s was the era of the 'power perfume'. 'Room-rocker' was the phrase coined for fragrances that filled a space with their intense olfactory vibration – leading to a ban in some parts of America for scents such as Giorgio Beverly Hills, out of a fear that these scents would dominate food aromas and flavours, spoiling the enjoyment of fellow diners. Landmark launches included Dior Poison, Calvin Klein Obsession, Guerlain Samsara, Chanel Coco and Givenchy Ysatis (all of which endure to this day) – and women who liked to make their presence felt helped them to achieve blockbuster status.

But, as ever, fragrance fashions mirror hemlines, from one extreme to the other. So the 1990s were all about understatement: cleaner, sheerer scents such as Issey Miyake's ground-breaking L'Eau d'Issey, which was created to look – and even smell – like water, with its crisp ozonic/woody notes. Then ck one, launched by Calvin Klein in 1994, heralded a return to the tradition of 'shared' perfumes – back to the time when fragrance didn't have a gender, but was simply worn because you loved the smell. (Though in this case, maybe the advertising, too.)

The millennium saw the rise of the 'niche' or 'cult' perfumer. We think of the years since the turn of this century as the most exciting phase in fragrance history since the innovation of synthetics opened up a world of possibilities to perfumers back in the late 19th century. The landmark? In 2000, a Frenchman named Frederic Malle (read more about him on page 86) launched his 'Editions de Parfums' collection – which announced the names of the 'noses' on the plain-and-simple bottles. And suddenly, a scent-loving public woke up to the notion that perfumery, like painting, music and photography, is another art form designed to delight our senses. The boundless creativity shown by independent perfumers since then has given mainstream perfumery a jolt – and resulted in new collections of exclusive scents, of daring limited editions, and the acknowledgment of gifted 'noses' whose involvement was once a secret.

And personally…? We can't wait to see – and smell – this next era in fragrance history, and everything that's still to come. Fully confident that before long, someone will have the technology, which enables us to smell a new launch via our iPhone before we flex our Amexes.

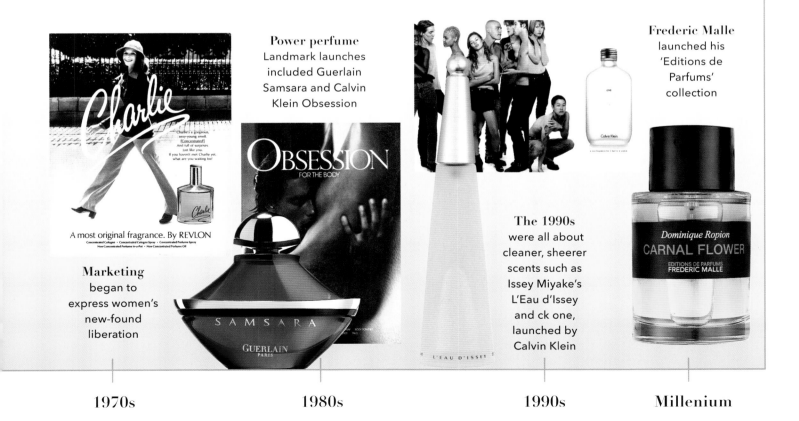

Power perfume
Landmark launches included Guerlain Samsara and Calvin Klein Obsession

Frederic Malle launched his 'Editions de Parfums' collection

Charlie

A most original fragrance. By REVLON

Marketing began to express women's new-found liberation

OBSESSION
FOR THE BODY

SAMSARA
GUERLAIN
PARIS

L'EAU D'ISSEY

The 1990s were all about cleaner, sheerer scents such as Issey Miyake's L'Eau d'Issey and ck one, launched by Calvin Klein

Dominique Ropion
CARNAL FLOWER
EDITIONS DE PARFUMS
FREDERIC MALLE

1970s   **1980s**   **1990s**   **Millenium**

a world of ingredients

Every fragrance is essentially a world in a bottle. The four corners of the globe have been scoured by botanists and perfumers on a quest for aromatic ingredients to tantalise, tease and tempt our sense of smell. And despite the rise of synthetic ingredients in perfumery, many plant-derived notes are still preferred for the richness that perfumers tell us that synthetics simply can't rival.

For many of the leading fragrance names, sustainability is a very real priority: without a secure supply, their very perfumes are at risk. But more than that: big fragrance suppliers have proved commendably keen to support the communities that depend on these precious harvests. With global business needing to be seen to 'give back' – and with all of us surely wanting to work for companies that are more than about just doing business, but also about doing good – there are some very interesting programmes in place which we hope are just a flavour of what's to come in terms of ethical and sustainable sourcing.

So let's go around the world in a dozen of the most 'important' notes...

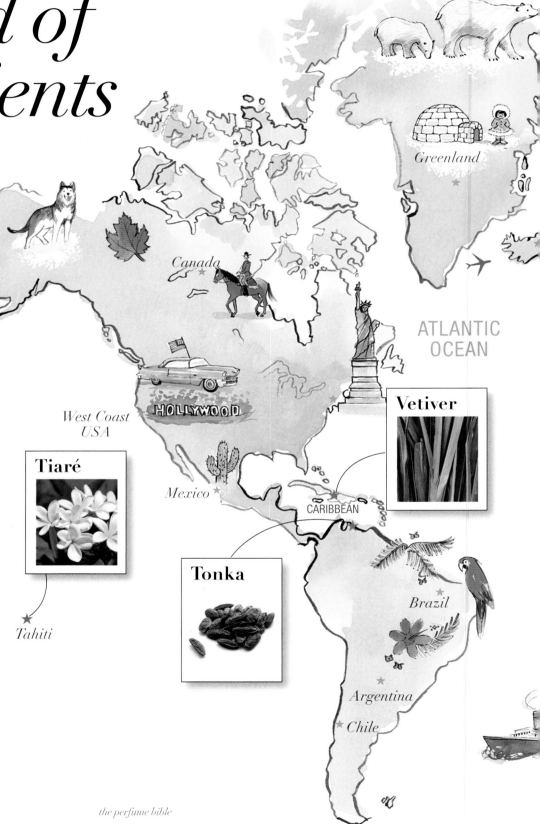

Greenland

Canada

ATLANTIC OCEAN

Vetiver

West Coast USA

HOLLYWOOD

Tiaré

Mexico

CARIBBEAN

Tahiti

Tonka

Brazil

Argentina

Chile

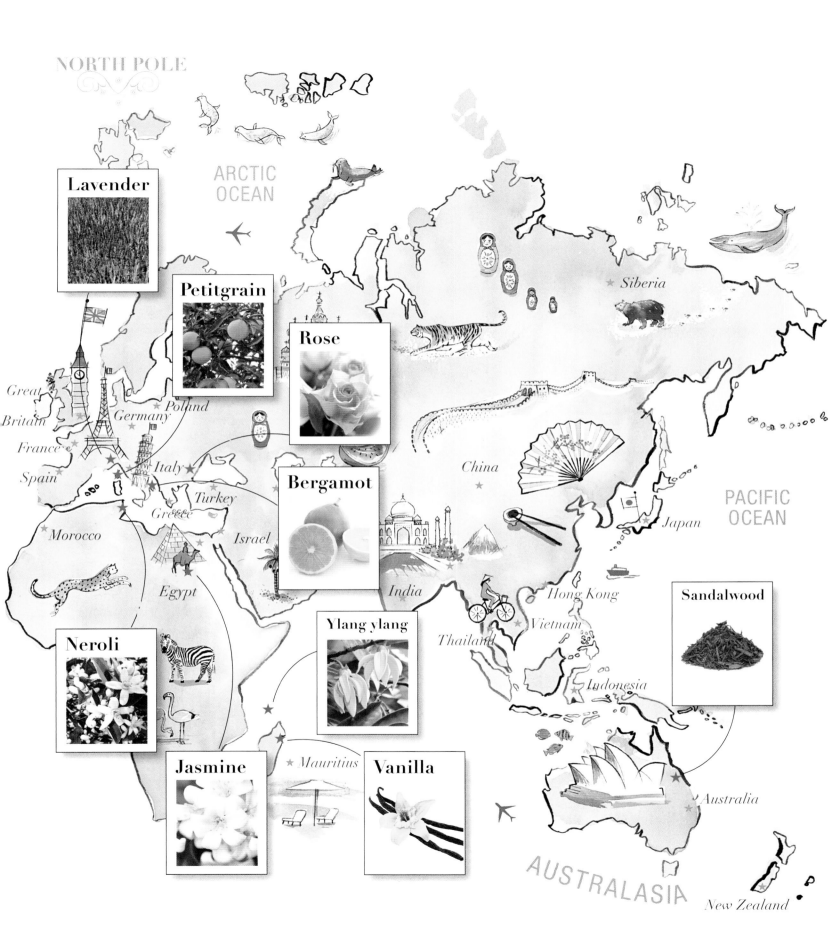

NORTH POLE

ARCTIC OCEAN

Lavender

Petitgrain

Rose

Bergamot

Neroli

Great Britain

France

Spain

Germany

Poland

Italy

Turkey

Greece

Israel

Morocco

Egypt

Siberia

China

Japan

PACIFIC OCEAN

Hong Kong

Vietnam

Thailand

India

Ylang ylang

Sandalwood

Indonesia

Jasmine

Mauritius

Vanilla

Australia

AUSTRALASIA

New Zealand

Bergamot

The very best bergamot – such a key, zesty top note in many fragrances – and downright essential for eaux de Colognes and chypre fragrances, comes from Calabria, southern Italy, which generates 90 per cent of the world's production. Zesty and sparkling, the fruit of the Citrus bergamia isn't harsh or acidic, but crisp and bright. It's one of the most widely-used ingredients, making even the richest and most opulent notes palatable.

Jasmine

Jasminum grandiflorum – which gives us the exotically sweet-scented jasmine oil – is grown in Morocco, India, Italy and China, with the most bountiful harvest coming from Egypt. As with rose, Chanel has its own jasmine fields in France, adjacent to the rose fields in a valley outside Grasse. This fragile flower needs to be processed swiftly to extract the precious oil – one of the most expensive ingredients in a perfumer's arsenal.

Lavender

Most of us can easily identify this wonderfully aromatic plant, even with eyes closed. France is still the heartland of lavender production; 60,000 kilos of lavender are said to be produced each year in Provence. Plants, though, are still vulnerable to a bacteria that weakens them; among other sustainability initiatives, the fragrance house Givaudan has been supporting production of healthy lavender plants, helping to protect this refreshingly scented ingredient for the fragrance industry.

It's all about the 'terroir'…

'Terroir' is a word more often used when talking about wine, or artisan foods. But fragrance ingredients, too, can be affected by 'terroir' - the location, even the very soil, in which they're grown. Amazingly, a 'nose' can often tell the source of a specific ingredient by smell alone - and it explains why perfumers are notoriously discerning about the sources of their ingredients, with the most fabled perfume houses monitoring production literally from field to flacon…

France is still the heartland of lavender production; 60,000 kilos of lavender are said to be produced each year in Provence

Neroli

The bitter orange tree – *Citrus aurantium var. amara* – gives us this exquisite airy, green, citrussy note, with its hints of honey and orange simmering underneath. Today, the best oil is said to come from Tunisia, although neroli is also harvested in France, Italy and even North America. As with so many key perfume ingredients, this white flower needs to be processed swiftly to retain its magic: the 'stills' are sited right next to the fields, to ensure that the process can take place as quickly as possible…

Petitgrain

Petitgrain – say it 'petty-gran' – comes, like neroli, from the bitter orange tree, but in this case, from the leaves and small twigs that are distilled a few weeks after the neroli harvest, to create a note that is woody, fresh, green and maybe a touch bitter, lending itself perfectly to masculine fragrances and also eaux de Colognes. It's harvested around the Mediterranean in particular, including Corsica.

Rose

Roses can be grown in many climates, but perfumers will tell you that the very best quality comes from Grasse, in the south of France, and from Bulgaria, where Guerlain perfumer Thierry Wasser tells us that no less than 200,000 people are involved in this annual harvest. In Grasse, Chanel is the only fragrance name to have its own rose fields: acre upon acre of sun-baked Provençale countryside, ablaze with pink for just a few precious weeks a year.

Sandalwood

For many, many years, most sandalwood came from India. But over-harvesting means that sandalwood has become endangered, with the few old trees that remain now mostly on private property, and many younger trees suffering from disease. Still, there's a happy 'next chapter' in the history of this sublimely soft and sensual base note: the true Indian sandalwood tree *Santalum album* can be cultivated successfully in Australia, where 25-year-old managed trees are now starting to produce high-quality oil. It is, however, very pricy – and only the finest perfume houses use the real deal.

Tiaré

Also known as 'monoi' de Tahiti, this hypnotic, heady, almost intoxicating ingredient makes its way into white floral scents and Orientals. The symbol of the island, it is worn as garlands and tucked behind the ear during special ceremonies and holidays – but the closest the rest of us get is dabbing a drop or two behind the ears, instead...

Tonka

This dark, shrivelled-looking ingredient (actually a member of the pea family) has appeared in many gourmand fragrances, as well as Orientals, giving a warm smoothness and reminiscent of caramel, almond and tobacco. Fragrance house Givaudan helps to support tonka bean farmers in the Caura Basin area of Venezuela through training in drying, processing and storing (among other things), in exchange for a commitment to preserve 88,000 acres of forest, and the animals and plants within that natural resource.

Tiaré is the symbol of Tahiti, it is worn as garlands and tucked behind the ear during special ceremonies and holidays

If you're interested in delving deeper into ingredients, there's a rather charming book – *The Scent Trail*, by Celia Lyttelton – which is the account of one woman's personal olfactory odyssey, as she embarked on a journey to trace the origins, history and culture of her favourite perfume elements. A fascinating read that we recommend, if you want to find out more about ingredients, their sources – and the romantic ways that those ingredients made their way into a bottle, and onto our skins...

Vanilla

So vital an ingredient for 'sexy' fragrances, this sweet, sensual note is extracted from the seeds of the dried pod of a climbing orchid-like plant that flourishes in Madagascar and particularly in the island of Réunion. Fragrance house Firmenich's sustainability team uses an enlarged, floor-sized Google map of Madagascar to determine how to protect the forest ecosystem, while helping farmers to plan vanilla crops.

Vetiver

It smells earthy – but vetiver's actually a deep-rooted grass, most widely grown on Réunion (where much of the vanilla crop also comes from) and Haiti. After the earthquake which devastated Haiti in 2010, fragrance producer Firmenich has been involved in a sustainability project, helping not only to improve agricultural methods and training, but providing better access to jobs, education, water, hygiene and nutrition. More generously used in men's perfumery, vetiver also makes its way into women's perfumes as a base note. (Guerlain, meanwhile, has its own sustainable vetiver project in Tamil Nadu.)

Ylang ylang

Another exquisite exotic, this tendrilled tropical flower that blossoms on a tall tree. So potent, so heady, so sensual – and also, so threatened by deforestation and erosion. International Flavors and Fragrances (IFF) is working in the Comoros Islands on reforestation programmes to preserve not only supplies of *Cananga odorata* but also the surrounding landscape, and to help improve the living conditions of the farmers who harvest this sublime ingredient, through clean water access and health programmes.

what the noses know

'A perfumer…needs more than a passably fine nose. He needs an incorruptible, hard-working organ that has been trained to smell for many decades, enabling him to decipher even the most complicated odours by composition and proportion, as well as to create new, unknown mixtures of scent.' So wrote Patrick Süskind in his extraordinary, unputdownable novel *Perfume*, which is a must-read for all perfume-lovers. And it's still the most perfect description of a perfumer that we've ever come across

Talk to perfumers – or 'noses' as they're known in the business – and it becomes obvious why they choose to make their living by making scents. Fragrance is a way of life for them; they aren't content to breathe in a scent, but very often they eat, drink, think and – yes – even dream about scents, too. And despite huge technological leaps in so many industries, fragrances are still fashioned in much the same way as they have been for centuries, with magic formulas concocted by gifted perfumers – those 'noses'.

Perfumers themselves don't always love that tag; as Jean-Claude Ellena, who now works in-house for Hermès, agrees, it's strange that a perfumer is referred to as a 'nose' when nobody would think of calling a composer an 'ear'. 'As an organ,' he points out, 'my nose simply performs a control function. I smell with my brain. It stores every scent and knows how to combine them; the perfumes I create originate in my head.'

A perfumer is able to summon up to 3,500 different odours, memorised by wafting scent-dipped, blotting paper mouillettes under the nostrils for hours, even days, until the fragrance (and its future possibilities) is registered. Bearing in mind that many of us, when asked to name an unidentified smell on a blotter, feel as if we're fumbling in the dark, it's some gift.

We couldn't be more pleased that at, last, that gift – and the extraordinary creativity of perfumers – is being more widely

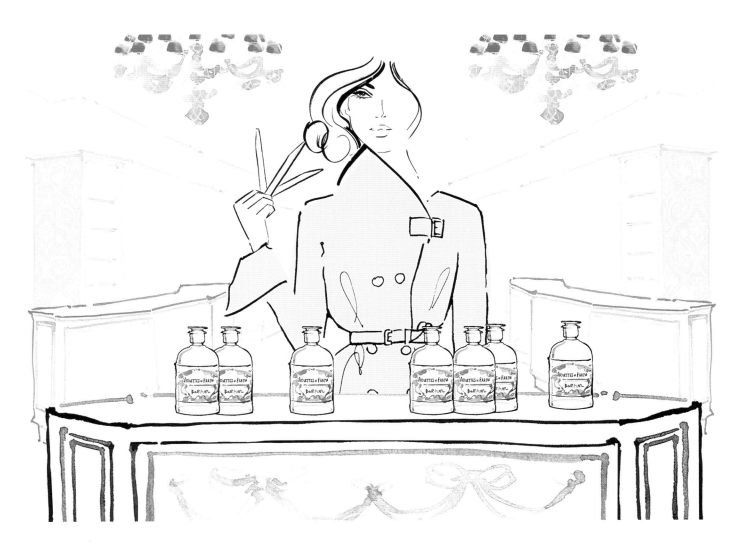

acknowledged and recognised as an art form in itself: in 2012, *The New York Times* 'perfume critic' Chandler Burr curated an exhibition at the Museum of Arts and Design, The Art of Scent, which firmly put perfumery up there with music and art itself – where we believe it belongs.

The highlight of our 20-plus years (each!) of working within the perfume industry has been the time spent in the company of some of the greatest perfumers on the planet: Jean-Claude Ellena (see left) and Christine Nagel (now at Hermès), Jean-Paul Guerlain, Jacques Polge and Christopher Sheldrake (Chanel), Mathilde Laurent (Cartier), Jacques Cavallier-Belletrud (now at Louis Vuitton), Karine Dubreuil (L'Occitane) and Francis Kurkdjian among others. (And we're delighted to be able to introduce many of those leading figures to perfume-lovers, at least in the UK, through subscriber events for The Perfume Society.)

One of the most acclaimed perfumers working today, meanwhile, is Thierry Wasser – the first non-family member to take up the role of perfumer at the legendary house of Guerlain. Initially, Swiss-born Thierry worked alongside Jean-Paul Guerlain – who he still regards as a father figure.

He is one of the few perfumers in the industry who control key ingredients right from the field where they grow though to the final product, to ensure that the quality meets Guerlain's exacting standards. Since 2008, during his time at Guerlain, Thierry has created several spins on Idylle, La Petite Robe Noire, Shalimar Parfum Initial, and each year's limited-edition Aqua Allegoria, among other creations.

We met with him at the staggeringly glamorous restaurant at Guerlain's Paris flagship boutique, Le 68, over a Shalimar tea (scented with cardamom, cinnamon, lavender and bergamot),

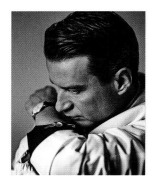

"

As a perfumer, it has been an eye-opener for me to realise that every decision to buy an ingredient has a direct impact on the livelihoods of many people, and it's so important to me to respect that

Thierry Wasser

and pastries, which are also confected (by Michelin-star chef Guy Martin) to evoke Guerlain fragrances…

What was your first encounter with fragrance?
'I must have been 13. I didn't really look my age, physically; I felt I looked as if I was about eight. A friend of my mother's used to wear Guerlain Habit Rouge. I wanted to make it mine, because I thought it was very manly. It was my first fragrance.'

How did you become a perfumer?
'I didn't know I wanted to become a perfumer – but so much of life is about encounters… I had an interest in botany, and in nature. And I started as an apprentice to a herbalist called Edmond Burri; he was the first man who believed in me. When you're a kid of 15, thrown out of school, you need that – and so initially I spent my Saturdays mixing up herb teas and pomades and syrups in that herbalist's shop. Then at 19, I wrote to the head of the Perfumery School at Givaudan, in my home country of Switzerland, which I thought would be fun. I had no idea I would love it so much.' (By 1987, he had graduated as a Fine Fragrance Perfumer with Givaudan in Paris, before moving on to Firmenich in New York.)

Was it scary, stepping into the perfumer's shoes at the house of Guerlain?
'I wasn't afraid, joining Guerlain, but of course it was an esteemed position to take up. We'd already got to know each other when I created two fragrances for the house, Quand Vient la Pluie and Iris Ganache. In 2008, I was approached to work alongside Jean-Paul Guerlain, and we were together in the lab for several years before he retired. What strikes me most is how long Jacques and Jean-Paul Guerlain kept at it (for more than 50 years each). As true masters, each of them managed to imprint their own style on the House. At the beginning, it was wonderful to be able to see Guerlain through the eyes of Jean-Paul, and I still have lunch with him once a week, on a Wednesday – not in a professional capacity, but because he really is like a father to me.'

What does your job entail?
'I spend a couple of days a week in my lab, working on fragrances. Tuesday is my "business day", because I sit on the Executive Committee, which means I get to see a complete picture of the brand, its history and its growth.

'I get to express my creative side in the lab, but I'm also in charge of quality control: every material that comes into the factory and everything that goes out as a bottled product is checked by my team – there are 11 of us involved in quality control, sourcing, buying. On Wednesday I'm at the factory all day.

'My job is different to my previous roles, because now I'm responsible for sourcing of the key ingredients for our fragrances, to ensure quality control and security of supply. The ingredients are so important: it's rather like making Champagne. The harvest can vary depending on the weather, so there's a level of uncertainty every year. What's wonderful about this particular job is the people; you're not just buying ingredients, it's a relationship. I am involved directly with the farmers who produce bergamot in Calabria, where they're now growing jasmine for us, too, in fields that have been replanted with what was a traditional crop. We have a project that is incredibly close to my heart in Tamil Nadu, where farmers are growing vetiver for us. I travel to Bulgaria for the rose harvest; the whole process of rose production involves 200,000 people, and Guerlain buys between 8 and 10 per cent of that harvest. As a perfumer, it has been an eye-opener for me to realise that every decision to buy an ingredient has a direct impact on the livelihoods of many people, and it's so important to me to respect that.

'In Tunisia, I am involved in the whole orange flower harvest – overseeing the workers, checking the flowers, weighing them and then supervising the extraction of the fragrance elements through old copper stills, which deliver a much better quality of oil than modern stainless-steels stills. I guess I'm maybe the only perfumer in the industry who is getting his hands dirty in this way, seeing that ingredient right through from the field to the finished product in the bottle.

'Another necessary part of my job is travelling to Brussels, occasionally, to ensure that perfumers have a voice when changes are proposed for laws that could affect the future of our industry. Around 20 per cent of my time is spent on the road; nobody knows about that – they think you're always in the lab, with a white coat on…'

How many fragrance ingredients do you work with?
'I have around 750 materials to work with – which is a lot. But as an exercise, I decided to recreate all the old Guerlain formulas myself, just so that I could smell them, to help me get inside the head of Aimé Guerlain, or Jacques Guerlain – fragrances which aren't available any more, because ingredients have been restricted through regulations, or simply because a particular style of scent has gone out of fashion. So sometimes I have just a tiny amount of something, and other times it's a kilo.

'I am incredibly fortunate to have the old Guerlain formula books at my fingertips, and to be able to go back and see where Jacques Guerlain wrote a note in the margin of Aimé Guerlain's formula, saying something along the lines of, "August 1940: because of the War, civet has become unavailable because the source is under German occupation, and has been replaced in the formula for X by X…"'

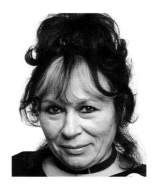

A perfumer can almost taste a scent. It fills up your nose but it can also give you the feeling of eating and drinking. And sometimes, you can even smell the fragrance you're working on in your dreams…

Sophia Grojsman, creator of Trésor and Calyx

At any one time, how many fragrances are you working on?

'I do between six to ten bespoke fragrances a year for private clients – roughly one every two months. But every year there is an Aqua Allegoria launch to create, new concentrations of existing fragrances – an eau de toilette or an extrait for La Petite Robe Noire, say – together with other launches for the future. And because of changes in regulations and safety guidelines, I sometimes have to reformulate a fragrance with slightly different ingredients, playing with the formula to ensure that so far as the perfume-lover is concerned, it smells exactly the same as it always has.'

Can you share an example?

'For instance, there have been restrictions on oakmoss because of a specific part of oakmoss that has been linked with sensitivity. Oakmoss is an incredibly important ingredient to Guerlain, most particularly for Mitsouko, which is one of our greatest treasures from the past, along with Jicky, L'Heure Bleu and Shalimar. Happily, fragrance ingredient producers have been able to "fractionate" oakmoss, to remove the allergen. But the challenge is that when you remove something from an ingredient, it leaves a "hole", and the fragrance won't smell the same; for a while, there were complaints about that, because the character of Mitsouko had definitely changed. I had the idea of adding a tiny touch of celery to the oakmoss, to complete it – et voilà: happy Mitsouko-lovers tell me that once again, their fragrance smells like it should.'

How long does it take to bring a fragrance to life from an idea?

'Around two years. Around 12 months to play with the idea, then polish it and modify it till everyone – and especially me – is happy. And then around another 12 months for stability tests, for compatibility tests (to ensure it works with the bottle); you put it in the oven and in the sun to check it doesn't change colour for instance…'

Do you have to be in a particular frame of mind to create?

'There may be noses who are like Tchaikovsky, a man who could compose when he was depressed – but I'm not like that. I need peace. I need joy. I have to have a drink from time to time and smoke a cigar.'

As a 'nose', does yours ever switch off?

'Yes, it really does. It's a question of paying attention; when I'm working, I'm absolutely focused on what I'm smelling. But off-duty? Not so much. On the way here, a big bus farted fumes in my face as I was crossing the Champs-Élysées, but I didn't find myself analysing what was in those fumes. That would be exhausting!'

There are said to be fewer perfumers than there are astronauts. Becoming a perfumer takes years of training and students must show true aptitude; initially, they generally undergo a series of 'odour evaluation tests'. If successful, the would-be 'nose' may be taken on as an apprentice (six years), or as a trainee at a fragrance supplier (Givaudan, Firmenich or IFF), or by one of the few perfumery training schools in the world. To be admitted to the Institut Supérieur International du Parfum de la Cosmétique et de l'Aromatique Alimentaire (ISIPCA) in Versailles, Paris's perfume school, a student must already have a degree in chemistry, biochemistry or pharmaceuticals.

Being a nose has its romantic moments, for sure – but rock-solid maths and chemistry are required to cope with the challenges of hundreds of formulations and reformulations (or 'mods', short for 'modifications'), which take place on the journey from concept to launch. Languages are useful, too; perfumery is an international profession.

And it isn't all about creating 'designer' perfumes for key brands: many perfumers spend the majority of their career creating fragrances for items such as laundry products, household cleaning must-haves and cosmetics (beauty products).

I am a lover of poetry. What would reality be without its poetic dimension? Even if you don't read poetry, it plays an important role in everyday life. I am a lover of fragrance, and fragrance is a form of poetry. It doesn't speak – but it gives so much…

Jacques Polge

FROM FIELD TO FLACON:
the making of a perfume

Almost since the dawn of recorded history, we've been looking to enhance – or maybe mask – our own natural smells through the use of perfumes. Initially, incense was used: it didn't just fragrance a room (or rather a tomb in Ancient Egypt), but the smoke would perfume clothing, too. (There are similar rituals in Arabia, even today: clothes are censed with 'fumigation' – washed, dried and then placed on a rack over a special incense burner.)

Most of the fragrance worn today, though, is in liquid form. A delicious alchemy of leaves, flowers, grasses, fruits, woods, resins and gums is generally blended with the synthetic ingredients, which gives staying power or helps 'diffuse' a fragrance when it's sprayed, or simply recreates in chemical form some of the elusive scents that can't be captured naturally. (Plants such as lily of the valley are incredibly shy about giving up their

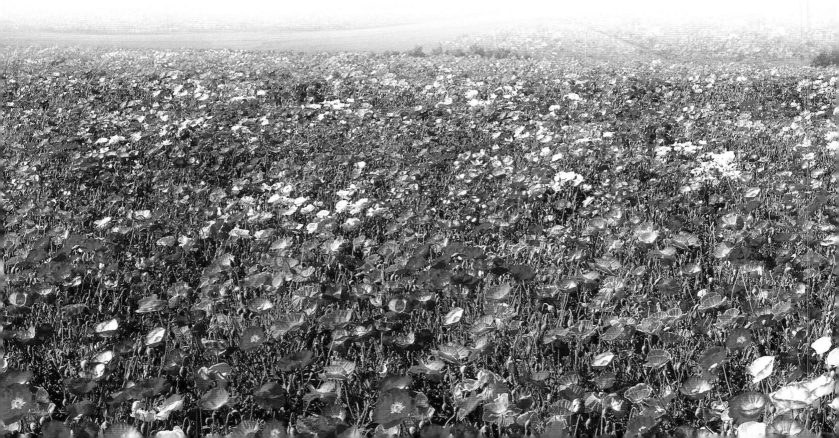

fragrance, so clever chemistry must come into play.) Here's how it's done...

Here's how it's done:

In the field Perfume ingredients are grown all over the world: roses in Morocco, Bulgaria and Grasse; sandalwood in Australia (which is taking over from India for environmental reasons, see page 55), vetiver in Haiti, bergamot in Calabria, in Sicily. All natural ingredients must be harvested at the optimum time, which is critical with flowers such as jasmine – pickers in Grasse are in the fields by dawn, and finished for the day by elevenses. Their bounty is then rushed to the factory for extraction before the fragrance dims. (In the case of Bulgarian rose, distillation may even happen right there in the field.)

Some perfume houses, such as Chanel, have exclusive contracts with growers to ensure consistent supplies of ingredients. Their jasmine and rose is grown (and rapidly processed) there.

Steam distillation Fragrant ingredients like roses, ylang ylang, eucalyptus leaves are placed in a 'still' (aka an 'alembic'), and steam is passed through the raw materials. The volatile fragrant compounds evaporate and condense, and pass into a second chamber. This allows for easy separation of the fragrant oils from the water, as the oil floats to the top of the 'distillate' and can be removed. The water left behind still retains some aromatic compounds, though; you might buy it as a 'floral hydrosol'. Rose water and orange flower water are created in this way, as a by-product from the production of more precious, pricy fragrant oils.

Enfleurage Once upon a time, particular kinds of flowers were layered between glass plates covered with highly purified, odourless vegetable or animal waxes. Freshly picked blooms – jasmine petals, for instance – were then spread across the wax and pressed into it, and over a few days or weeks (depending on the botanical ingredient used) would disperse their scent into the fatty mixture. The depleted flowers were then removed and replaced with a fresh harvest of just-picked petals, and the process repeated until the greasy mix became saturated with fragrance.

At that point, the 'enfleurage pomade' – the fragrant, fatty oil – was washed with alcohol to separate the extract from the fat. (That was generally used to make a rather delectably scented soap.) Once the alcohol had evaporated, an essential oil was left, for use in perfumery. However, as you can imagine, the whole process is unbelievably expensive, and nobody does it any more. The word enfleurage, though, is still used – but generally refers to the process of solvent extraction. It's a way less romantic but far more reliable (and inexpensive) method of ending up with the same thing.

Solvent extraction Fragile flowers such as hyacinth, linden blossom, mimosa, narcissus, tuberose and jasmine just can't handle the heat of steam distillation. Instead, essential oils can be extracted by solvents such as hexane (mostly), or dimethyl ether – and the resulting

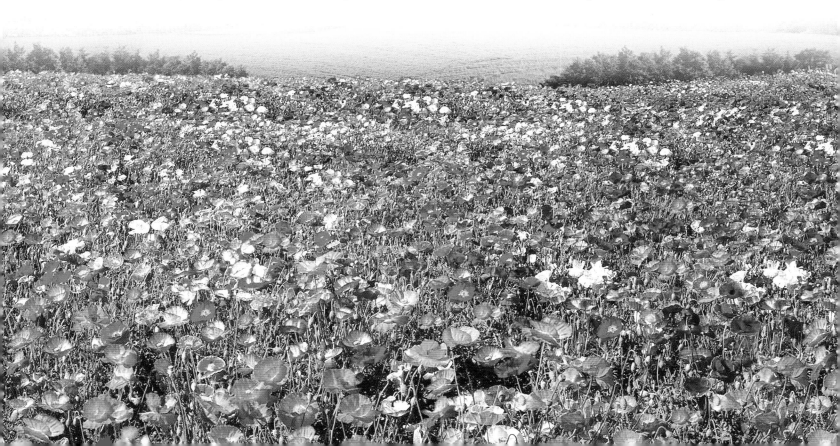

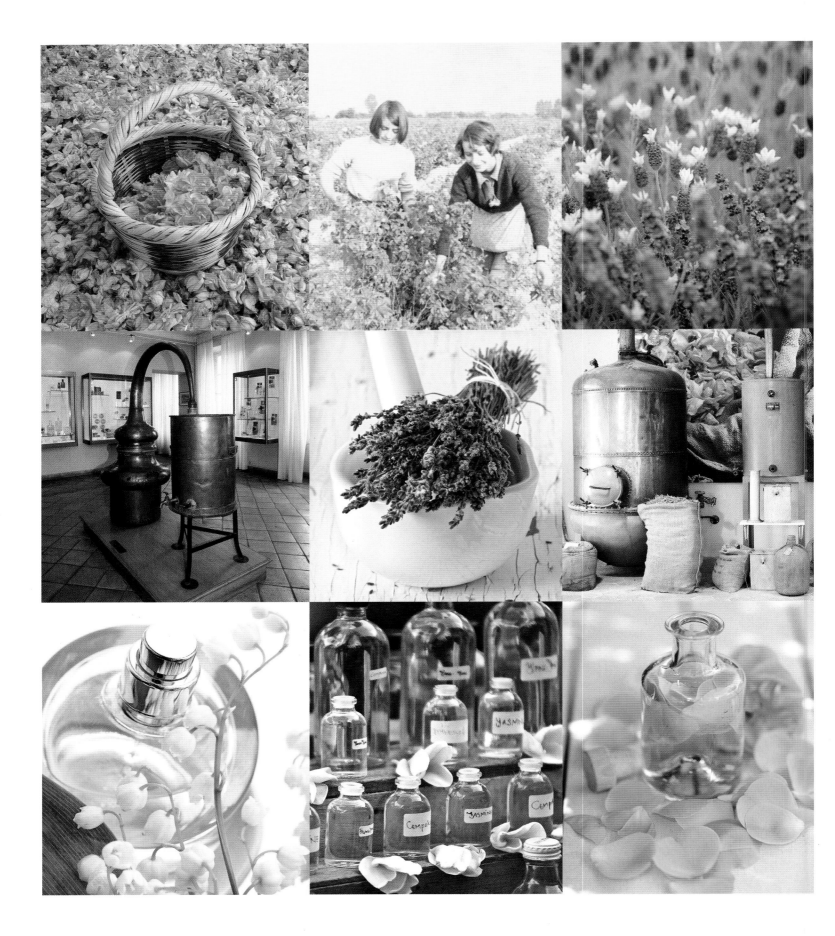

essential oil is very close to the natural fragrance of the material used. The harvested flowers are layered in giant metal perforated drums and washed repeatedly with the solvent. This dissolves everything that can possibly be extracted from the plant: non-aromatic waxes, pigments and the precious, highly volatile aromatic molecules.

Not surprisingly, the liquid then has to be filtered – but that means the solvent can then be recycled over and over again. The waxy mass that's obtained from the process – similar to the process of enfleurage – can contain as much as 55 per cent volatile oil (in the case of jasmine), and is known in the industry as a 'concrete'. (It's pronounced the French way – 'con-kret' – which sounds a lot more glamorous than the similarly-named building material.)

This could be used in this form as a solid perfume, but generally the waxy concrete is warmed and stirred with alcohol (usually ethanol) to make an 'absolute'. During the heating and stirring, the waxy concrete breaks down into tiny globules, which partly separate out – but to ensure the job's done thoroughly, the solution may be agitated and frozen at very low temperatures, then cold-filtered for absolute purity.

Absolutes are the priciest, most precious of perfume ingredients and are more concentrated than essential oils.

Supercritical fluid extraction Very high-tech name, very high-tech process, although it's a bit easier to get your head around when you know it's also called 'CO_2 extraction'. We're not going to blind you with the science bit: just to say that in this case high-pressure carbon dioxide gas is used as a solvent. As this is a low-heat process, the fragrant compounds often closely resemble the smell of the original material. Ingredients derived in this way are known as (yes!) CO_2 extracts.

We love the idea that our fabric conditioner may have been produced by the gifted individual who also created a bestselling fragrance

Cold pressing/expression We've all dug our fingers into a citrus fruit and enjoyed the 'burst' of essential oil which that produces from the skin. Well, scale that up and you've got the process of cold-pressing: machines score the rind, then capture the resulting oil. Citrus oils can also be captured by steam distillation, but those in the know maintain that cold-pressed oils are much more vibrant.

All of these ingredients are then mixed with other aromatic compounds, and diluted with alcohol. This is where the genius of the 'nose' comes in – and to read about their role, see page 56.

The role of the fragrance house… Only a handful of perfume brands – Chanel, Dior, Louis Vuitton, L'Occitane, Cartier, Jean Patou and Hermès – have their own in-house perfumers. Other brands generally turn to one of the 'fragrance houses', which employ perfumers who may work on a wide range

of fragrances – as well as household products such as shampoos and even cleaning materials and washing powders. (We rather love the idea, personally, that our fabric conditioner may have been produced by the gifted individual who also created a bestselling fragrance. Do give your Lenor another sniff when you're next loading the tumble dryer and muse on that.)

A brand – perhaps a designer brand, or even a well-known luxury house such as Mont Blanc pens or Bentley cars – will often brief several of these fragrance houses, soliciting submissions for a planned launch. It's basically a competition. The 'customer' (ie the brand) generally writes the brief – target age bracket, male/female/shared, the season it's to be worn in – and often accompanies it with a 'mood board' montage of images designed to conjure up a vision, or feel, in the perfumer's mind.

These fragrance houses are the unsung heroes of perfumery, if you like. Their names are almost unknown to the average perfume-wearer: IFF (International Flavors & Fragrances), Givaudan, Firmenich, Takasago and Symrise. (There's also a house called Robertet, based in Grasse – the very heartland of traditional French perfumery – which specialises in natural ingredients, and is a go-to fragrance house for brands with a more natural bent.)

There's another important role within a fragrance house: the 'evaluator'. Their names are mostly unknown, too – yet their noses are as finely tuned as those of perfumers. When the brief, or 'fragrance request', arrives via the sales department, the evaluator steps in. She figures out which perfumer/s would be right for the job and communicates the brief – including maximum cost of the final 'juice', restrictions on materials, who that all-important final customer might be and deadlines.

The perfumer – with his or her encyclopaedic knowledge of raw materials – writes the fragrance formulas. These are sent to the compounding lab, where they're mixed and blended. Alcohol is added, and the samples are sent back to the evaluator. She smells, and smells again, seeking the best 'fit' for the client. Will it play well with a younger market? Is it sexy, as requested? Is the gardenia – which the client wants to take centre stage – dominant enough? And thus begins a to-ing and fro-ing; sometimes, a perfumer will work on dozens of different 'mods' (as they're known – short for modifications) before the evaluator decides it's right to pitch to the client, who's likely to be smelling submissions from several houses. And even when the deal's been clinched, there may be many more modifications along the way before someone says, 'enough, perfect'.

As Lauren Salisbury, who works as an evaluator in the US, explained in her article 'How many hands touch your bottle of perfume?', for the terrific Bois de Jasmin blog: 'An evaluator carries a great deal of responsibility for the success of a fragrance project – and all the joys and burdens that responsibility bequeaths. An evaluator must have the nose, the love of perfume, and the knack of following her gut, just as perfumers do. She must be brave and bold enough to dream up her own ideas and share them, but modest enough to listen to others, as well'. The career of an evaluator, Lauren explains, 'is both thrilling and exhausting. The best parts are evaluating and smelling everything out there on the market; sharing and brainstorming ideas with other evaluators; offering an idea to a perfumer and seeing the spark of creative excitement in his eyes because he "gets it" and may be onto something… and then winning a project'. One of the worst parts, she adds, 'is being the bearer of bad news when telling a perfumer that the ideas didn't work or didn't smell right

You put your heart and soul into coming up with what you think is the best possible fragrance for a client, but there's no runner-up, no second place. You either get the commission, or you're out. It can be heartbreaking

Francis Kurkdjian

(nobody likes to be criticised!), or that the project was lost.'

So yes, perfumers themselves have to be pretty thick-skinned. They often do lose out to 'noses' from other fragrance houses, who win the 'beauty pageant' of submissions. As renowned 'nose' Francis Kurkdjian observes, 'You put your heart and soul into coming up with what you think is the best possible fragrance for a client, but there's no runner-up, no second place. You either get the commission, or you're out. It can be heartbreaking.' (Fascinatingly, these fragrance houses set sales targets for their leading perfumers to hit each year, in dollar/euro earnings for the fragrances they've created. If they have a 'hit' for a big customer, they may get to work on a more 'niche' – which can sometimes translate as less commercial/more adventurous or avant-garde – project, for a different client.) For more about the life of the nose – and to learn about their boundless creativity – see page 56.

Once a fragrance house lands the deal to produce a scent for a brand, they take care of production, too, in their own factories and facilities – diluting the precise blend of aromatic ingredients on the 'spec' to the correct concentration with alcohol/water. (For more on fragrance strengths, see page 20.)

Again, only a tiny number of the larger perfume houses control and manage their own production from start to finish, let alone from field to flacon – although many 'niche' and independent perfumers do blend, dilute and hand-fill (and hand-label) their own bottles, artisan style. But it's not for the romance of it; with global players to do business with – including some of the most famous designer names on the planet – the large fragrance houses simply aren't set up for the small runs that are all a just-starting-out perfumer can stretch to, as they build their marque…

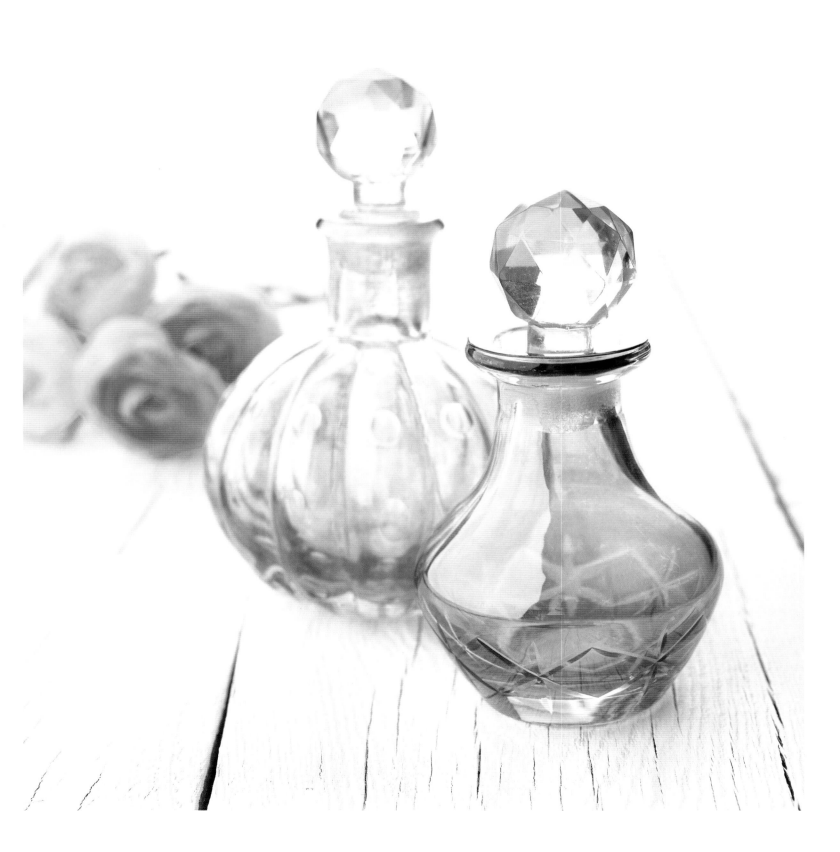

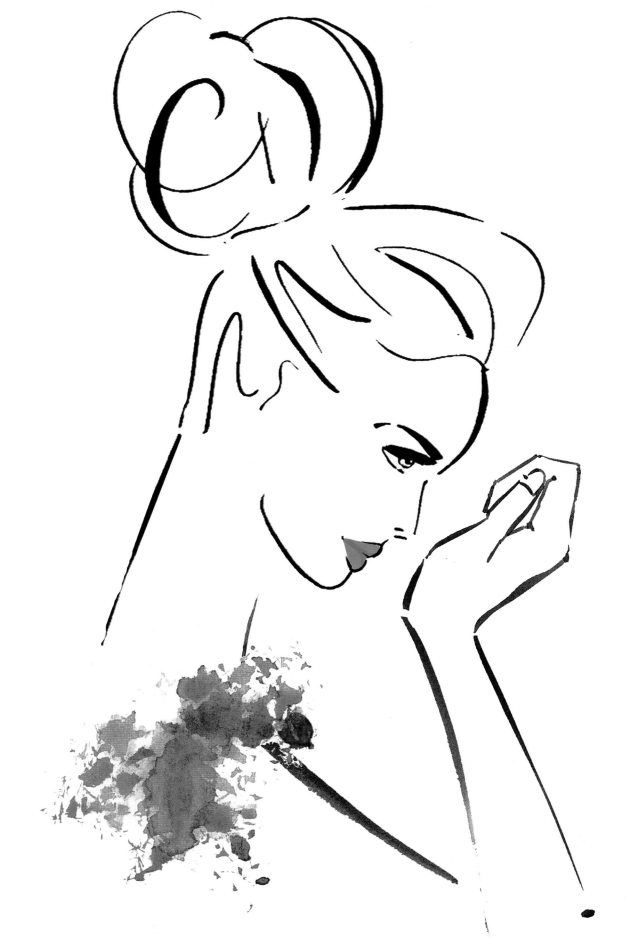

"

As a perfume doth remain
In the folds where it hath lain
So the thought of you, remaining
Deeply folded in my brain,
Will not leave me: all things leave me;
You remain…

"

From 'You Remain' by Arthur (William) Symons

natural ♡ *synthetic*

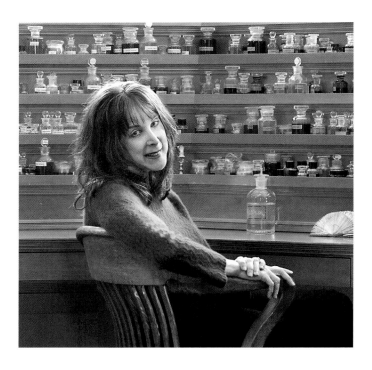

Mandy Aftel is the author of some of our favourite-ever fragrance books and brilliant at conjuring up exotic smells through words in fabulous reads such as *Essence & Alchemy* and *Scents & Sensibilities*. She's also terrific at conjuring up fabulous fragrances themselves: a self-taught perfumer, Mandy has chosen to work with naturals as her field of expertise, with her own Aftelier range, which has been shortlisted for several Fragrance Foundation Awards. Mandy is also founder of the Natural Perfumers Guild, which was started in 2002 to raise awareness of botanical fragrances

Now, we know from years in this business that the word 'natural' does something to people. Maybe it's because, for the first time in history, we are predominantly 'living in our heads', out of touch with the earth and even our senses for much of each day while peering at screens (of one kind or another).

'Natural perfumery', then, has a sort of get-in-touch-with-the-seasons vibe to it – almost as if at one sniff, it will reconnect us with the earth and the seasons. Perhaps for that reason, all the major perfume houses like very much to make a big thing of the natural elements in their fragrances: the rose and jasmine, bergamot and neroli, frankincense and patchouli. But in reality, there are no mainstream fragrances at all that incorporate nothing but naturals; they're mostly blends of naturals and synthetics, in varying proportions.

And there's a reason for that: however glorious, in their natural state those pure botanical essences present a perfumer with various challenges – which this accomplished perfumer talked about, here, when we spoke to her from her perfume studio in Berkeley, California…

Just what exactly is natural perfumery?
'It's the art of creating beautiful luxury fragrances, using only natural essences. These botanical essences come from flowers, fruits, leaves, roots and barks. Natural essences, unlike their synthetic counterparts, contain minute trace elements which change their character – hence why Moroccan rose smells different from Bulgarian rose or Egyptian rose.'

How did you get into natural perfumery?
'I started working with naturals around 20 years ago and I fell in love with them, simple as that. I'm someone who truly follows my nose in life, going towards what I find interesting. After a long career in psychotherapy, I decided to write a novel and made my main character a perfumer. I knew I had to smell some of the materials that perfumers work with, and I couldn't believe their complexity and how they touched me.'

What do you love about it?
'An inescapable aspect of smelling a natural perfume is the way that it connects you to the smells of the natural world, in the same way as a walk in the forest, cooking a delicious meal or harvesting plants and flowers from your garden. There is a richness to knowing that the essences you're inhaling played such a rich part in human history. After all, we smell not only with our nose but with our mind.'

What are the challenges you face as a natural perfumer?
'You can't simply throw a bunch of natural ingredients together and get a great perfume, any more than you can with synthetics. But the biggest difference is how they behave on the skin, and you have to be ready for that.

'Natural perfumes don't broadcast their presence and only last about two hours on the skin. In contrast, the thing that allows perfumes to endure from morning and night, and to be perceived from across the room, is the presence of synthetics. Perfumes that purport to be all-natural, but last all day or have a sillage of 3 metres (10 feet) are not truly from botanical sources.

'Purely natural ingredients don't have that staying power, and won't "project" as far; it's a more intimate experience. Certainly naturals do cling to the skin, but pretty much everything I make is still designed to be touched up during the day. I sell jewellery for that exact purpose, so that you can wear your perfume and re-apply it over and over again – which is one of the most pleasurable parts of wearing a perfume, after all…'

Are men and women drawn to different types of naturals?
'Funnily enough, my experience is that almost always men turn out to like florals. I once did a class at the Apple headquarters in California and all the men went for florals. By contrast, there are lots of women who are drawn to deep, earthy notes like patchouli and vetiver. It's important to remember that really not so long ago, there were no distinctions between male fragrances and female fragrances. And I don't think there should be; everyone should be free to wear what they love.'

Do you have specific favourite ingredients?
'They change all the time as I discover new materials. Recently it's been tiaré, an amazingly exotic oil from Tahiti. Then I came across some eucalyptus absolute: it's sharp and camphoraceous and I'm just loving the challenge of trying to incorporate it into a fragrance without it becoming medicinal and overwhelming. I absolutely love ambergris because of its mythical status: it is simply washed up on the shore, a waste product from the whale's digestive system – what could be more rare and precious than that? I completely love my materials and I spend a lot of time and a complete fortune sourcing them, and then turning them into artisanal fragrances.'

Should we shop for natural fragrances differently?
'They're definitely best experienced on the skin, rather than smelled in the bottle or on a perfume blotter. They have a unique interaction with your body chemistry, blossoming on the skin. These perfumes smell unique on each person, which is part of their allure and magic. The best way is to put some on the back of your clean, un-fragranced hand. Allow the alcohol to disperse, or it'll diminish your ability to smell the perfume. Close your eyes when you smell the perfume and focus on that initial aroma. Take note of the complexity, texture and shape of the scent. Notice how it has changed. Smell again after ten more minutes and then again after half an hour. This will give you a good reading of the evolution of the perfume on your skin.'
www.aftelier.com

plant a perfume

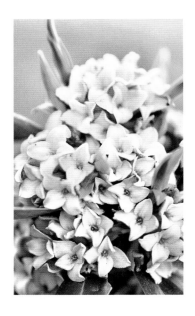

It's obviously not quite possible to replicate the fragrance of Chanel No. 5 simply by planting roses and jasmine next to each other. (We wish.) But (tulips aside) we've never quite seen the point of planting an unfragranced plant when there's something aromatic out there that could fill the space equally gloriously – and fill the air with its scent at the same time

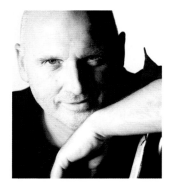

So we asked
Sam McKnight to recommend his favourite scented plants for the garden. Though better known as a session and catwalk hairstylist (his Chanel shows are legendary), Sam is an avid gardener with a deep love of scent and smell.

Depending on where you are in the world, some plants will flourish better than others – but these are all uttlery divine ways to perfume a yard or a whole garden…

Daphne odora

'I'm not sure why nobody's ever captured the spicy, almost incense-like scent of this plant in a perfume; it's sublime. It takes a little while to get going, but fills a whole courtyard with the fragrance of its pink, clustered flowers. The variety *Daphne odora* '*Aureomarginata*' has green leaves with a creamy edge to them, and is gorgeous, and *Daphne bhoula* 'Jacqueline Postill' is another favourite – with, if anything, an even more exquisitely rich scent.'

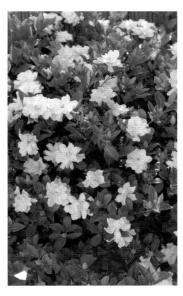
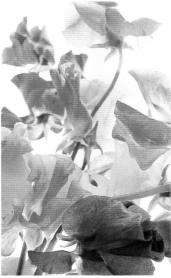
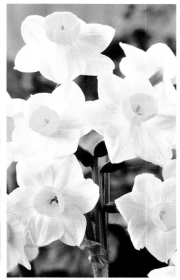
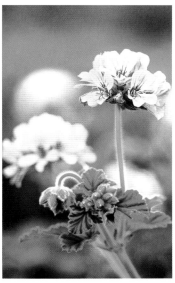

Gardenia

'This was one of Coco Chanel's favourite flowers, and it has a very "Chanel" feel to the exquisite, creamy-white blossoms, which are wonderful against the dark green shiny leaves. It does well in places like California and in tropical locations – plants can grow to eight metres high! – but in colder climates it's a terrific tender houseplant that can be put outside in summer. It likes an acid soil, so be sure to get the right compost, which mustn't be allowed to dry out. You'll only get a few blooms at a time, but that's enough to fragrance a whole room.'

Lathyrus odoratus

'What's a garden without sweet peas…? I can't imagine summer without them, but not all sweet peas are created equal and there are some definite scented must-haves, such as "Painted Lady", "Black Knight", "Lord Nelson" and "Matucana", which probably has the most spectacular aroma of all. As the flowering season progresses, the stems of sweet peas tend to get shorter – and obviously, longer stems look better in a vase. The trick, I've found, is to keep sweet pea plants really well watered and then the stems stay really long, making for the most perfect, delicately-scented cut flower.'

Narcissus 'Avalanche'

'Narcissi are always a cheery sight in spring; I sometimes miss the first of them when I'm doing the catwalk shows for autumn-winter, but it's fantastic to return home to this early hint of the warmth to come. Many daffs don't smell, but this yellow-centred white narcissus has a wonderfully rich, complex scent that fills a room if you can bear to cut them for the home.'

Pelargonium 'Attar of Roses'

'Pelargoniums are scented geraniums; unlike bedding geraniums, which have garish flowers, these tend to have dainty blooms, but wonderfully fragrant leaves. For many people, rubbing an almost-furry pelargonium leaf between their fingers whisks them straight back to childhood because of the scent – which can range from lemony through to a beautiful rose geranium fragrance, here. Smelling this is exactly like sniffing a bottle of rose geranium essential oil…'

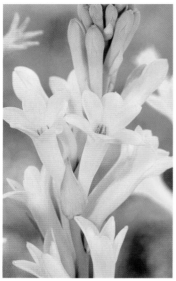 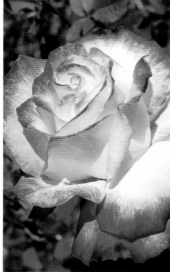 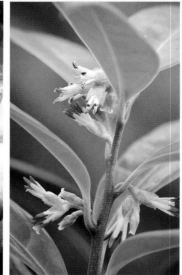 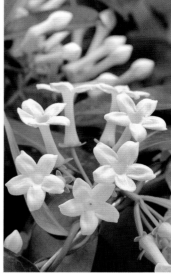

Polyanthus tuberosa

Tuberose is a classic fragrance ingredient; Piguet's Fracas is dominated by this fragrance (as was Madonna's debut scent, which was inspired by her mother's Fracas). The complex, intoxicating scent of tuberose really does smell like an actual perfume in its own right; a bit headache-y for some people, but others (including me) love it. In warmer zones tuberose can be planted outside in well-drained soil (tuberose hates having wet feet), but the bulbs can also be grown very well in a greenhouse, where the fragrance will billow out through the open windows on a warm day.'

Rosa 'Double Delight'

'This gets its name from the fact that it's beautiful to look at – creamy white, with pink-tinged edges that get deeper and darker as it ages – and just as beautiful to smell. I've heard that Evelyn Lauder, who was heavily involved in the creation of many Estée Lauder fragrances, grew this on her Manhattan rooftop and had it incorporated as a perfume note in the perfume Intuition. There are many, many different scented roses, but this is a gem.'

Sarcococca hookeriana var. humilis

'This shade-loving fragrant sensation is a great "beginner's" plant because it's so easy to grow. Small plants take a while to clump up, but the added bonus is they're evergreen. The tiny, almost fluffy flowers blossom during the colder months and the intense tropical flower scent wins out over almost any other winter bloom. One of these in your garden is a great invitation to get out there and breathe some fresh, sweet-scented air on even the gloomiest day.'

Stephanotis floribunda

'This is also known as Madagascar jasmine, waxflower or Hawaiian wedding flower. In colder climates it's generally grown as a houseplant, but is wonderful on a garden table on a terrace during summer months; they definitely need warmth and plenty of light to flourish. The incredibly highly fragranced waxy flowers contrast with the dark green foliage and as it's a climber, you'll often find it twined around a circular piece of wire when it's sold as a potted plant. I've smelt some wonderful stephanotis-based perfumes, but the "real deal" is quite intoxicatingly gorgeous.'

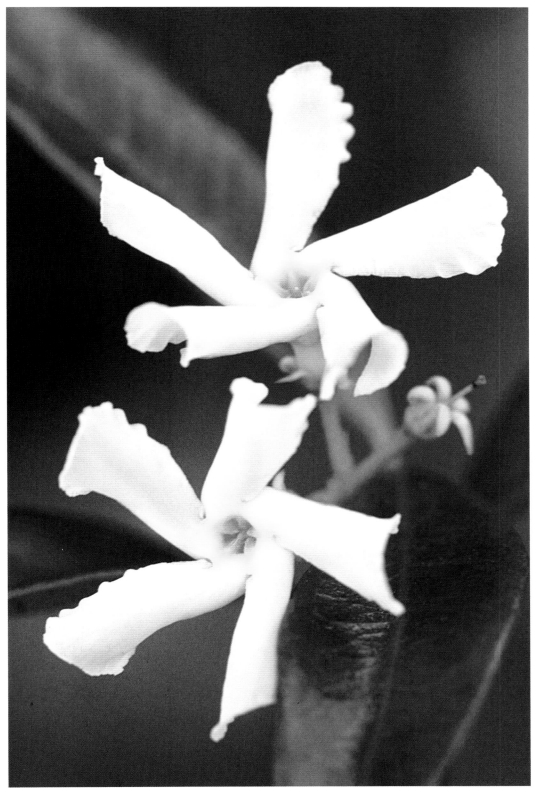

Trachelospermum jasminoides

'I love the smell of jasmine, but outside of hot climates it's not the easiest plant to keep happy. So I'd recommend this alternative: an evergreen, shiny-leafed, climbing "star jasmine", which likes full sun or dappled shade and lots and lots of water. Provided it's not in a windy spot, it's trouble-free and heaven-scented – just like jasmine itself.'

> **"**
>
> *I'd recommend this 'star jasmine' as an alternative to the usual jasmine variety*
>
> **Sam McKnight**
>
> **"**

collecting perfume art

Some extraordinary artists, illustrators and photographers have created imagery for perfume advertising over the years – and thanks to the internet, it's easier than ever to track them down…

From Dali to René Gruau, leading names have lent their artistic talents to advertising scents. Gruau's drawings for Dior are among our absolute favourites – Miss Dior, Diorissimo, Diorella, as well as Rouge Baiser lipstick. Gruau 'moonlighted' for other fragrance brands, too, including Balmain. And ads for Balmain, Lanvin and Schiaparelli come pretty close, in our book. Then, of course, there are the beauties photographed for Estée Lauder's wonderful 'lifestyle' adverts in the 1970s (we admit: we tore them out and Blu-Tacked them to our walls), and Chanel's legendary names – from Catherine Deneuve to Carole Bouquet via Inès de la Fressange and, more recently, Nicole Kidman and Vanessa Paradis. The iconic No. 5 bottle was also painted by Andy Warhol (Chanel produced a limited-edition box with the drawing on the outside that is very collectible now).

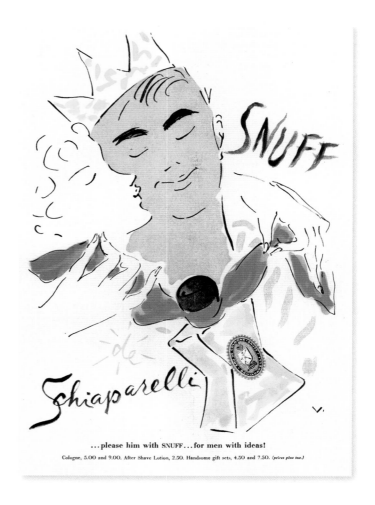

...please him with SNUFF...for men with ideas!
Cologne, 5.00 and 9.00. After Shave Lotion, 2.50. Handsome gift sets, 4.50 and 7.50. (prices plus tax.)

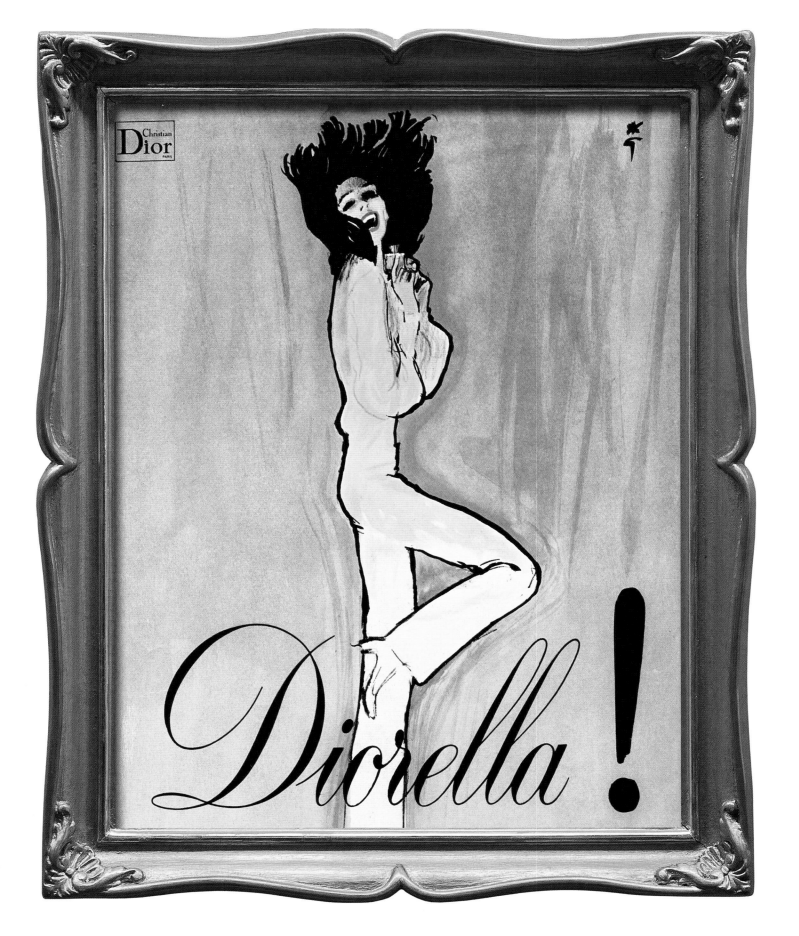

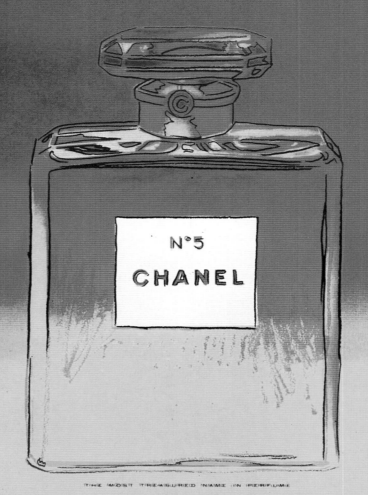

N°5
CHANEL

THE MOST TREASURED NAME IN PERFUME

CHANEL

> *Gruau's drawings for Dior are among our absolute favourites – Miss Dior, Diorissimo, Diorella... The iconic No. 5 bottle was also painted by Andy Warhol*

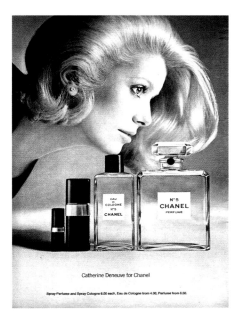

Catherine Deneuve for Chanel

Spray Perfume and Spray Cologne 6.00 each, Eau de Cologne from 4.00, Perfume from 6.50.

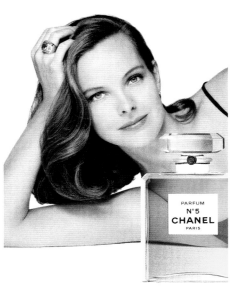

PARFUM
N°5
CHANEL
PARIS

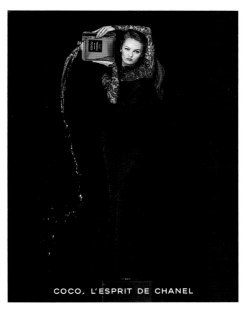

COCO, L'ESPRIT DE CHANEL

A wonderful website where you can trawl through the decades and swoon over some of these historic ads, meanwhile, is www.vintageadbrowser.com, on which they're divided into decades. It's like a window on the social changes of the 20th century, as expressed through perfume imagery and slogans.

And if you'd like to have them in your life (and your home or office)? Etsy and eBay are good sources for vintage perfume advertising, while Etsy also features portfolios of many contemporary illustrators who incorporate fragrance bottles in their work. The British site www.vintageinprint.co.uk generally has iconic perfume ads for sale, but it's also worth trawling through vintage magazines in secondhand/antique stores; if you can't bear to rip out the pages (truly, we can't any more), they can of course be scanned (and then even printed onto canvas).

If you really want to continue the perfume theme, Google 'perfume bottle fabric' and various results will come up. And for more inspirations of gorgeous homes incorporating fragrance in the décor, visit www.houzz.com and put 'perfume bottles' in the search box. The most stylish perfume decoration we've ever seen, though, has to be a Hermès 'perfume bottle' silk scarf from the 1980s in a gorgeous gilt frame. (The scarves themselves do come up on eBay too, albeit pricily.)

Do also look at David Downton's fabulous coffee table book *Masters of Fashion Illustration*, written by our very favourite illustrator of all, and showcasing work by everyone from Erté to René Bouché. Only a smattering of perfume ads, but gorgeous anyway.

perfume, bottled

Is it wrong to buy a fragrance because you like the bottle?
Not necessarily, if you don't mind having it as an ornament.
But fragrance brands aim for you to fall in love with the whole
'package': the bottle, the 'juice' (maybe the colour of that
'juice', too) – and even the advertising

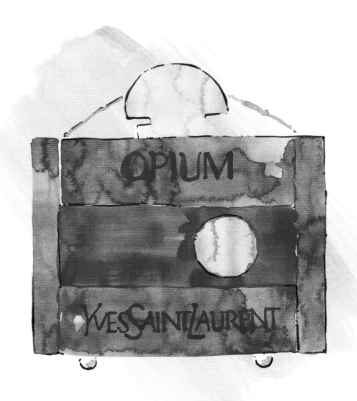

The design of the flacon is definitely an all-important element of a fragrance, for many brands – and the art of bottle creation is a fascinating world in itself. On a fragrance counter crowded with hundreds of new scent launches each and every year, a simple glass container may not cut it any more in the crowded arena of the perfume hall.

As you may have noticed, the design of many perfume bottles has become evermore extravagant and bold in recent years. 'There are endless rows of counters of fragrance and you have a millisecond to catch a customer's eye,' observes one fragrance retailer. So, the cap of Marc Jacobs's Dot is a large butterfly. Plastic daisies adorn the lids of (yes) Daisy, with different colours used for various 'spins', which have followed that bestseller. Viktor & Rolf's second scent, Bonbon, comes in a huge pink glass bow. Glowing, by Jennifer Lopez, was designed to light up for 15 seconds, when sprayed. The creativity seems boundless…

Pierre Dinand is one of the legends of bottle design responsible for that creativity: Givenchy Ysatis, YSL Rive Gauche and Opium, Chanel Eau Sauvage and Lancôme Magie Noire are among the many he's crafted over a more-than-50-year career – all classic designs that have withstood the test of time. His very first bottle was Madame Rochas, which was released in 1960 – and Pierre never looked back, even though that very first commission almost came about by accident.

'I was working in 1958 and 1959 as Art Director in an advertising agency, which had clients involved in luxury goods – including Champagne, Cognac and fashion. One of the companies, Marcel

Rochas, liked my new graphic approach, and knowing of my architectural study background asked me if I had any ideas for the shape of a new perfume bottle that would carry the name of a beautiful woman, Hélène Rochas. That was new to me but very challenging. I decided to spend time with Hélène Rochas, falling in love with her. I got inspired by a collection of antique perfume bottles she had at home. The problem was to produce industrially something that was originally handmade. It worked and was an enormous success. I was immediately requested to create bottles by many other fashion designers – Pierre Balmain, Pierre Cardin, Christian Dior, Yves Saint Laurent. Each time I thought this would be the last and I would have to design some other things, but it kept going, increasing demands from all over the world...'

Inspiration, for a designer like Pierre Dinand, can strike in many ways – and poses some serious technological challenges. In the early 1960s, as his website (see Directory) reveals, Dinand had a dream of locking Paco Rabanne's Calandre into a metal frame. Back then, metal was almost impossible to use in a perfume bottle context, but Pierre found a brand new material used in the car industry. Once galvanised, it could be metal plated – and the frame looked like real metal.

Later, in the 1980s, Pierre was playing golf when the ball smashed. 'Inside, there was this weird material used for the stuffing. It looked like frosted glass but wasn't. It had a depth of contrasts that no other material could offer.' That was one of the inspirations for Obsession, but the rich amber colour came out of a meeting with Calvin Klein himself. 'Calvin told me he liked black and white, but I wasn't about to design another No. 5. I went to his house, which overlooked Central Park West in New York. In one room he had an antique tortoiseshell collection. That gave me the colour for Obsession. He had a collection of Tibetan stones, which gave me an idea for the shape…'

But the process of bottle design has changed as fragrance has boomed. Once upon a time, says Dinand, 'I used to work closely with the perfumer: Guy Robert for Madame Rochas, Edmond Roudnitska for Eau Sauvage, Michel Hy for Calandre. But it's different now; many different perfumers compete (for a commission) and I don't know the fragrance at the start. Still, I spend time with the noses, and try to exchange our views on the project. It's always better that the bottle and the 'juice' are worked together.'

For some 'niche' perfumers, though, the focus is most definitely on what's inside the bottle, rather than that bottle. And having a plain bottle hasn't held some of the smaller brands back at all. Rule-breaker that he is, Frederic Malle – the man who brought those 'noses' out of the lab and trumpeted their names on fronts

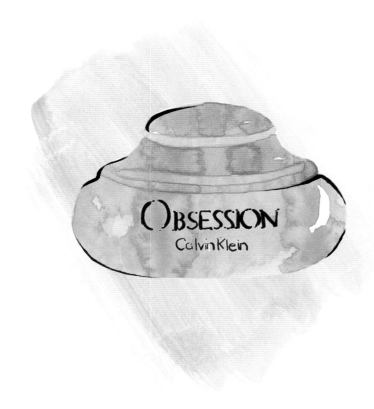

of bottles (see page 86) – chose a relatively understated flacon, with a plain black cap and label, for his scents. The same is true for many 'cult' brands, for purely practical and financial reasons: they can't afford to commission special bottles – when they're starting up, certainly – so must buy 'off-the-shelf'. But by doing that, they're also sending out a message in that bottle: judge me by the 'juice', not by appearances.

But in general, we do think that the world's a little unfair on perfume bottle designers, whose names often go unacknowledged when a fragrance is launched. In the case of many contemporary creations, the bottle is as key an element of the fragrance's success as the smell itself – and is often the first thing we fall in love with, at first sight.

Isn't it time – as is happening with the 'noses' – to allow perfume bottle designers to step into the limelight and take a bow? We'd say so…

In all seriousness, we'd like to see a move towards more 'refillable' bottles, in the style of Thierry Mugler's Angel and Alien, which can be replenished at what must be the world's most glamorous 'filling station'.

collecting vintage perfume bottles

This can be a wonderful pursuit. And with so many designs out there, from hand-painted glass decanters to Art Deco moulded figurines with Bakelite stoppers, it's no surprise that it has become a popular hobby. But for bottles from the important manufacturers – vintage Chanel, Baccarat and Lalique crystal flacons – there's serious competition on the internet. And at auction, too: in 2006, a shell-shaped frosted glass bottle containing a pearl-shaped bottle of Trésor de la Mer, designed for Saks Fifth Avenue by René Lalique in 1936, reached $216,000 at auction in New Jersey. (It was bought in 1939 for just $50 and the fragrance itself was long gone…)

Sometimes, just sometimes, you may catch a trace of the scent from times gone by when you snap up a vintage perfume bottle on eBay, or stumble upon one in a charity shop. But for the true connoisseur, this isn't about the perfume; it's about the container itself.

As perfumer and collector Roja Dove (creator of Roja Parfums) explains, 'the scent itself is irrelevant'. (Even in sealed bottles, it evaporates and oxidises with age.) 'Quality crystal glass bottles from Lalique or Baccarat were actually made in their thousands as soon as branded perfumes became a competitive area in the 1920s,' Roja observes. 'What collectors are looking for is interesting bottles for perfumes that flopped, launched only as very limited editions or – better still – that never got off the ground at all.' Then, says Roja, 'rarity value kicks in. And it's enhanced if the bottle is sealed and in the original box.' (Roja's own collection is seriously impressive, and much of it was displayed at Harrods's Perfume Diaries exhibition a few years back.)

For most of us, perfume bottle collecting is just a bit of fun rather than a serious investment. But if you do want to dip a toe into this whole fascinating area, you may want to check out the US-based International Perfume Bottle Association (www.perfumebottles.org), which showcases hundreds of bottles online and has links to many interesting sites devoted to bottle collection.

If you want to explore perfume bottle design in all its glory, we recommend *Glamour Icons: Perfume Bottle Design* by Marc Rosen, one of the world's most renowned bottle designers, who has designed for Burberry, Elizabeth Arden, Karl Lagerfeld and more, and has won seven 'FiFi' Awards (as the Fragrance Foundation Awards were called until recently). *Glamour Icons* is filled with images and anecdotes about the creation of his own designs, but also some of his 'vintage inspirations', including the Nina Ricci crystal dove bottle designed by Marc Lalique, Louis Süe's classically austere bottle for Jean Patou Joy and the amazing 'face' bottle by Hattie Carnegie for her signature scent.

> 66 *look for interesting bottles for perfumes that flopped, launched only as very limited editions or that never got off the ground at all… then the rarity value kicks in* 99

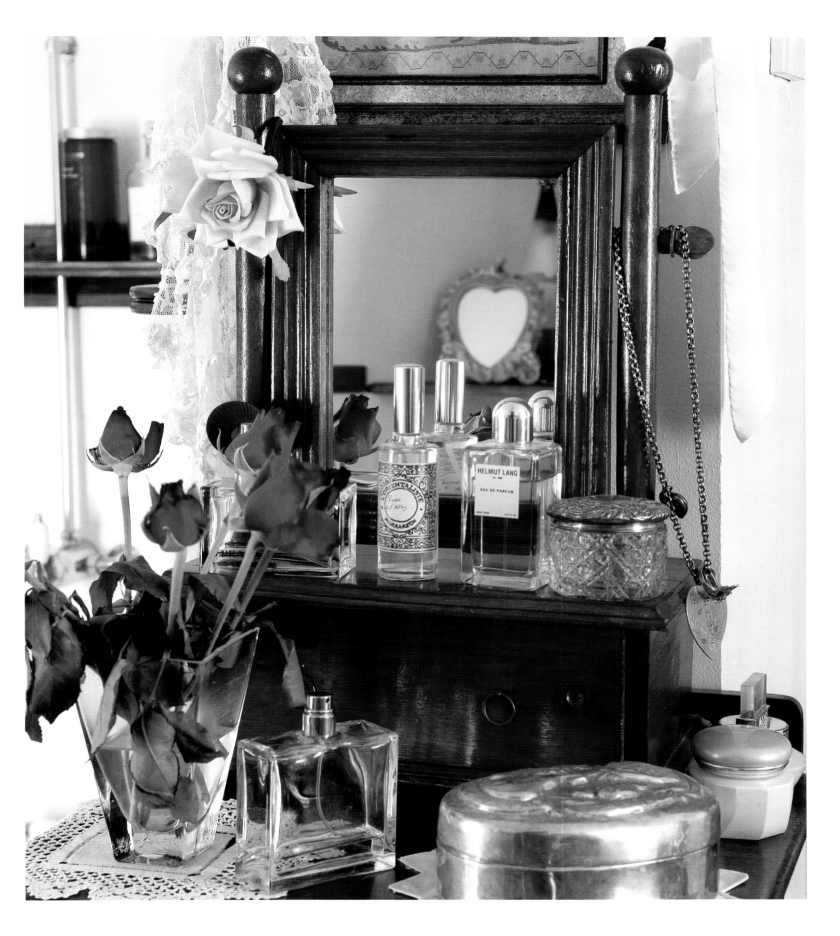

small(ish) is BEAUTIFUL

The MOST exciting thing has happened in perfumery in the last decade. Almost from out of nowhere have come dozens of truly talented independent perfumers, who are beckoning scent lovers away from the mainstream towards the enticing, intriguing, sense-tingling world of 'niche' fragrances

Some of these new brands are 'family affairs'; others are perfumers 'moonlighting' from their days jobs – and others still are brands founded by individuals who simply couldn't find what they were looking for to delight their senses among existing scents and set about commissioning perfumers to decant their dreams into bottles.

And we're loving this shift towards seeking out more daring, different, individual smells – definitely not the type of scents you'll find on the high street. There are thousands of these perfumes to explore; you'll mostly find them in smaller, independent perfumeries (some have their own stand-alone boutiques) – though larger stores are waking up to the perfumistas' passion for the extraordinary creativity of these niche perfume houses, too, and inviting those small brands in to be showcased in more 'traditional' perfume halls.

The reason for the creativity of these independent names is simple. Big launches need to be 'crowd-pleasers':

they're often researched and focus-grouped to the nines – which generally eliminates anything really daring and different. These rising stars can listen to their own instincts, maybe try a couple of things out on a friend – and that's as far as the 'focus group' goes. (You'll also discover that very few of these creations are overtly targeted at men or women, doing away with some of the traditional scent 'stereotyping'.)

The internet has also played a part in this revolution: not so long ago, it just wasn't viable for a teeny-tiny perfumer to launch a signature brand. Now they can do so in a tentative way, dipping a toe in the market with a basic website of their own, sometimes even hand-filling bottles to order (and very often wrapping the parcels and taking them to the Post Office themselves!).

Some of those listed here may yet prove to be the Guerlains or the Cotys of the future, but for now, they're still 'cult' finds, and every single one of the names below is worth taking time to sniff out…

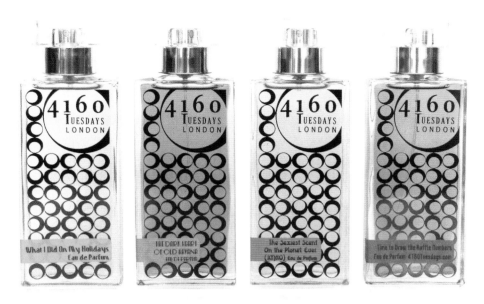

4160 Tuesdays

Sarah McCartney is a quirky, witty perfumer: though not formally trained, she did qualify in maths and sciences, knows what she likes – and has turned a hobby into a flourishing business. A dedicated collector of vintage perfumes, all her creations tell a story – and have accordingly intriguing names: The Lion Cupboard, Sunshine & Pancakes, Urura's Tokyo Café. And why 4160 Tuesdays? 'Because that's how many Tuesdays we have in an 80-year-old lifespan. So let's use them to write, think, make and do lovely things. Or if that sounds great but you don't have time, to buy lovely things other makers have put together.' We'll echo that. PS Sarah also runs some fascinating workshops you can check out on her website.

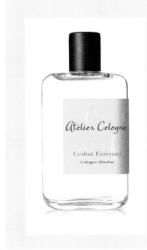

Atelier Cologne

A romantic tale, this: 'The trigger for Atelier Cologne comes from our encounter, our love for Cologne and our own love story,' says co-founder Sylvie Ganter, who set up this turbocharged Cologne brand with Christophe Cervasel, now her husband. Their idea was to create fragrances with the airy freshness of Colognes yet the richness of eaux de parfums. There are now more than a dozen Atelier Cologne creations to explore, boutiques in Paris and New York, and their Orange Sanguine – an absolutely sparkling whiff of blood orange, jasmine and tonka – won a FiFi Award (the Oscars of fragrance).

By Kilian

Kilian Hennessy has a luxury pedigree: his grandfather was the famed Cognac-maker whose empire now resides under the LVMH (the 'H' is for 'Hennessy') umbrella. Growing up in that world, Kilian went on to do a programme in communications and language studies, writing his thesis on 'the semantics of odours in the search for a common language between gods and mortals'. Crikey. Not surprisingly, each of the fragrances (now nudging 30 in number) tells an interesting, often intellectual tale (with names such as Forbidden Games, Good Girl Gone Bad, The Lotus Flower and The King Dragon) – and they're all exceptionally enthralling fusions, too, created with renowned noses including Calice Becker and Alberto Morillas. BTW, we very much like the idea that the exquisite, classic black bottles are refillable: there ought to be more of this 'eco-luxe' approach in perfumery.

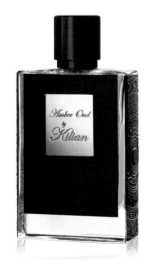

The focus has always been on quality materials rather than expensive packaging, and several 'editions' have gone on to become contemporary classics

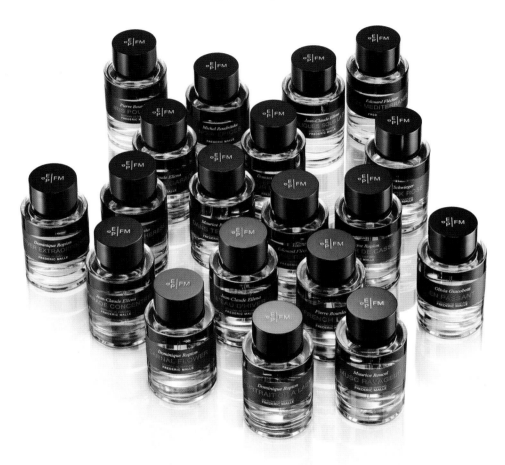

Editions de Parfums Frederic Malle

Frederic Malle isn't a perfumer – but he's changed the course of perfumery by offering some of the world's top 'noses' the chance to create the scent they'd always dreamed of, acknowledging them by trumpeting their name on the label. The focus has always been on quality materials rather than expensive packaging, and several 'editions' have gone on to become contemporary classics: tuberose-y Carnal Flower (by Dominique Ropion), Lipstick Rose (Ralph Schwieger), Musc Ravageur (Maurice Roucel). There are Frederic Malle boutiques in Paris, and shops-within-a-shop in leading department stores. Go. Smell. Enjoy. (And worship, in our case.)

Grossmith

Grossmith is one of England's oldest perfume houses, founded in the City of London in 1835. But although loved and worn by royalty (Grossmith was awarded Royal Warrants by Queen Alexandra and the Royal courts of Greece and Spain), and handed a prize at the Great Exhibition of 1851 for perfumes and essential oils, the brand became dormant in 1980 until founder John Grossmith's great-great grandson, Simon Brooke, brought it back again just a few years ago in 2009, relaunching delectable, nostalgic (and gloriously-named) classics like Hasu-no-Hana, Phul-Nana and Shem-el-Nessim ('the scent of Araby'). These have now been joined by some equally wonderful contemporary Grossmith creations: a lovely story, lovely scents.

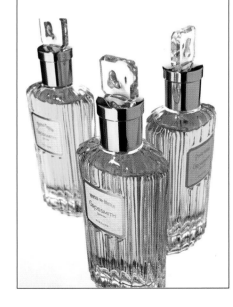

Heeley Perfumes

A (Yorkshire-born) Englishman and philosophy graduate based in Paris, self-taught in the art of traditional French perfumery (he's a designer by profession), James Heeley launched his first fragrance – the minty zoosh of Menthe Fraîche – in 2006. Originally, he worked with professional perfumers; now, James creates himself (while continuing to work as a brand and product designer) – and the results are often unexpected: Bubblegum Chic really does smell like a big pink bubble of Hubba Bubba chewing gum, while we're big fans of Hippie Rose, carefree and wild, with lots of harking-back-to-the-60s patchouli and incense in the base.

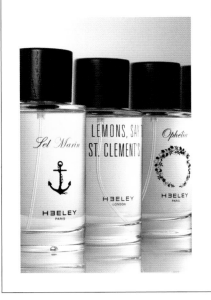

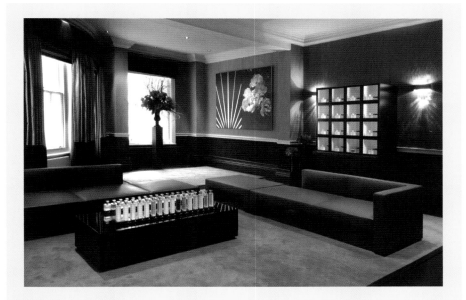

Illuminum

Illuminum rose to global fame almost overnight when the Duchess of Cambridge (formerly Kate Middleton) wore the brand's exquisitely opulent floral White Gardenia Petals for her wedding. Though the fragrances (more than 30 of them) are now more widely available internationally, surely the most enjoyable way to discover the collection is by embarking on a 'Sensory Journey' with one of Illuminum's in-house 'Sensory Guides' at their Mayfair Fragrance Lounge: a treat for the senses as he or she helps to edit down the collection based on your current scent faves, breathing each new offering from an upturned glass. Trust us: it's like 'a spa for the nose'…

Jardins d'Ecrivains

Something completely original, this: the fragrances (and candles) in this French line, from artistic director and photographer Anaïs Biguine, take their inspiration from writers and literature. Anaïs began by making candles, and got interested in the living spaces of writers when visiting the garden of Victor Hugo's home in Guernsey with her daughters. George Sand, Oscar Wilde, Virginia Woolf's Orlando and Colette's character Gigi have all now been captured in a bottle: it's a real delight to close your eyes and allow your imagination to transport you to their imagined spaces. (Do check out the fantastic travel candles in the range, too.)

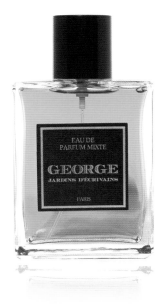

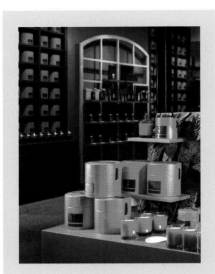

Jovoy

Jovoy is a store in the heart of Paris; a treasure trove of niche fragrances from around the world (as well as France), calling itself (unofficially) 'Embassy of Perfumes'. But Jovoy is also the name on a collection of glamorously packaged fragrances – some new creations, some vintage and some made 'for the mistresses of the Paris of the Roaring Twenties': in other words, 'opulent fragrances for women who wanted to be seen'. François Hénin is the charming Frenchman who's dared to rescue Jovoy from oblivion; previously, he spent years in Vietnam working in the essential oil industry and his passion for perfumery twinkles flirtatiously through every single Jovoy creation.

Juliette Has A Gun

There aren't many perfume creators who previously drove racing cars: Romano Ricci competed in France's famous Le Mans 24-hour race. But it was probably inevitable that he'd find his real calling in the world of fragrance: his great-grandmother was couturier Nina Ricci, while Romano's grandfather Robert created Nina's legendary signature scent L'Air du Temps. Romano persuaded perfumer Francis Kurkdjian to let him work alongside him – and after this 'apprenticeship', in 2006, launched the first fragrance under his innovative, elegant, albeit quirkily-named label. (Why so? 'Armed with her perfume, the Shakespearian heroine goes wild…') Our particular favourites are Romantina and the critically acclaimed Lady Vengeance.

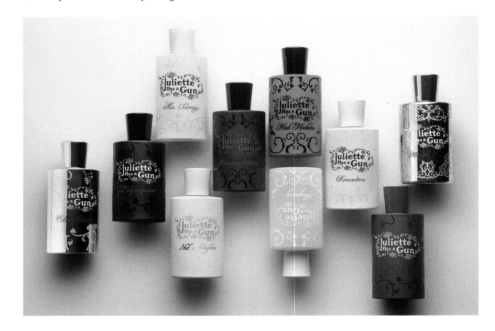

Londoner

Rebecca Goswell is a brand creator, trend predictor and creative director who worked with many of the world's most influential beauty brands before launching her own collection of fragrances, each inspired by a London postcode (and district): SE1 (echoes of London's spice wharfs), EC2 (traditional enough to be worn by a City gent, with its citrus, lime, grapefruit and juniper), N6 (a modern chypre), and so-feminine, nod-to-vintage W1X. To capture the essence of London's most colourful zones, Rebecca worked with her friend and fourth-generation perfumer François Robert, who happens to be based in the UK.

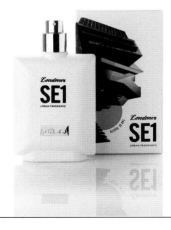

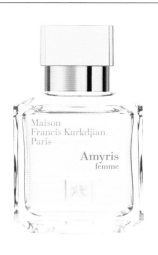

Maison Francis Kurkdjian

Regarded as one of the top three perfumers in the world, former ballet dancer Francis continues to work in mainstream commercial perfumery (think: Elie Saab, Narciso Rodriguez for Her) alongside producing extraordinary fragrances under his own name since 2009. They brilliantly conjure up feelings as well as scents: Aqua Universalis, one of our favourite Francis masterpieces, 'was inspired by the feeling of freshness: not the smell of fresh, but that feeling when you get into clean sheets in bed, in a hotel or at home'. There are several stand-alone stores, and this is a coveted brand for independent perfumeries around the world. Not at all precious about perfumery, Francis also offers scented bubbles for children, as well as the most wonderfully fragrant laundry products: your lingerie will never have smelled so good.

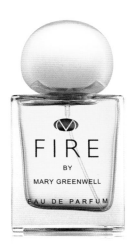

Mary Greenwell

Mary Greenwell is the globally renowned make-up artist who's channelled her lifelong passion for perfume into a very exciting collection of scents, working alongside perfumer François Robert. It makes sense: fragrance was always the last finishing touch Mary applied to her supermodels, giving them confidence for the camera. Her debut creation, Plum, is a quintessential chypre: super-sophisticated, super-feminine, super-sensual – and deserves still to be bewitching people in 100 years' time, we say. Her more recent creations – Lemon, Fire and Cherry – are no less interesting. A rising star and a lovely woman.

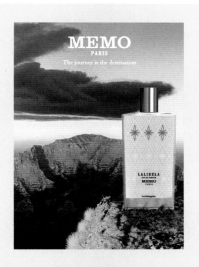

MEMO Paris

In common with Atelier Cologne, there's a couple behind MEMO: John and Clara Molloy (he was formerly an executive with L'Oréal and LVMH, and Clara was a writer). Avid travellers, they had the idea to create a brand that captured olfactory memories from their voyages: MEMO's simply short for 'memories'. Acclaimed perfumer Alienor Massenet creates what's in the bottles – which are all lavishly decorated with different designs in gold. The bestselling fragrance, mysterious rose Lalibela, is also our favourite, named after the Christian city in Ethiopia where angels are said to have come down from heaven to build 12 churches in a single night. Others are inspired by Ireland (Irish Leather) or Burma (osmanthus-rich) and named after the country's lake Inlé.

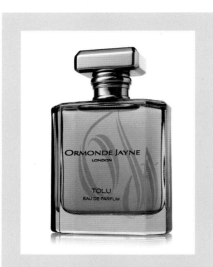

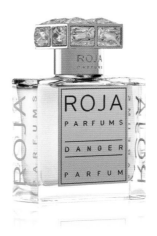

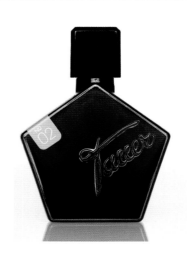

Ormonde Jayne

Linda Pilkington's Ormonde Jayne was one of London's pioneering niche perfumery lines, and her two boutiques (one in Mayfair, one in Chelsea) attract international scent-lovers in search of something different. We love her explanation of how she comes up with ideas: 'I get inspiration from absolutely anything. I might smell flowers on a beach in Mombasa, or see beautiful colours on a dress and think: "Hmmm, I could use that somehow."' Like MEMO's, Ormonde Jayne's fragrances are almost invariably triggered by her global travels, and we find the Four Corners of the Earth collection especially delicious (rich, decadently luxurious powerhouse floriental Tsarina is simply sublime).

Roja Parfums

You've almost certainly seen Roja Dove quoted as an expert on fragrance: his knowledge, having worked at Guerlain for many years, is encyclopaedic. (And his personal collection of vintage fragrances and bottles is probably unrivalled in the world.) After leaving Guerlain he first opened an exquisite Haute Parfumerie boutique in Harrods, and since then Roja has gone on to create his own line of perfumes, often using super-costly ingredients (and with price tags to match). He's managed to secure some very provocative names for his daring creations: Scandal, Risqué (read our review on page 142), Unspoken, Innuendo, Mischief, Danger and Reckless. We suggest you dare to try them for yourself.

Tauer Perfumes

A chemist by trade, Andy Tauer's a self-taught artisan perfumer who initially launched his line as a one-man business without giving up the day job. A charming and quiet Swiss-based man, much loved by perfumistas and bloggers, Andy thinks of his distinctively bottled creations as 'fragrant sculptures' – and they never fail to intrigue. There are several collections: Classics, Collectibles, PentaChords (which embody a 'less is more' philosophy of perfumery) and Homages – with especially 'precious' ingredients. We're enamoured of Le Maroc Pour Elle (warm spicy-rose, it really does conjure up the souk) and the bonfire-esque Lonestar Memories, in particular. The blog on his website is also an enjoyable 'follow', as an insight into a perfumer's mind.

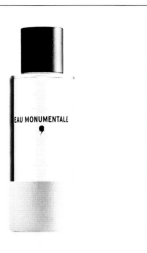

Thirdman

Thirdman's 'shareable' fragrances are as minimalist as the chic bottles, focusing on a handful of ingredients – and all (so far) are Cologne-esque. (Our top pick is the crisp, fresh citrus-aromatic Eau Monumentale, with its woody dry-down.) The man behind this deliberately enigmatic brand (with its cool silhouette) is Jean-Christophe le Greves. Formerly a creative director from the luxury goods world and now based at International Flavors & Fragrances in New York, he worked with IFF perfumers to create scents that are 'simple and streamlined, abstract yet familiar, and unlike any of their predecessors'. Unusually, it's recommended to keep Thirdman fragrances in the fridge, to turbocharge their refreshment even further…

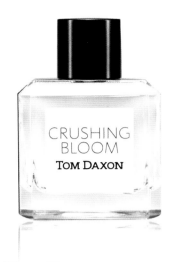

Tom Daxon

Tom's something of a perfume 'prodigy'. Though only in his early twenties, Tom explains that he's been 'surrounded by fragrance from birth': his mother Dale Daxon Bowers was creative director at Molton Brown for over 30 years, he grew up sniffing everything new that the brand launched (and lots it didn't), and often travelled with Dale to meet perfumer Jacques Chabert. On leaving university, there was nothing Tom wanted to do more than create his own fragrance line, and today, Chabert – and his daughter Carla – work with Tom on the beautifully-bottled line. Particular knockouts include rich Cognac-inspired VSOP, frankincense-powered Resin Sacra, and aromatic green Salvia Sclarea.

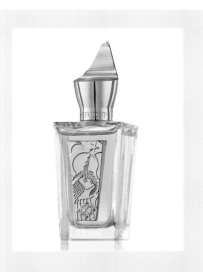

Xerjoff

The founder and creator of this Turin-based brand is Sergio Momo, who had a vision of 'luxury beyond compare' for his brand. (Xerjoff – say it 'Zer-joff' – was a nickname given by his Croatian grandmother.) Only the highest quality ingredients make it into what is now a massive range of over 50 fragrances using 'old-world artistry'. These are definitely luxe fragrances, presented with flair in bottles showcasing Italian craftsmanship: the Shooting Stars collection, for instance, comes in etched glass flacons with heavy gold caps, in a silken pouch – all of which contributes to making choosing your Xerjoff a very 'VIP' experience.

a bespoke fragrance:
THE ULTIMATE LUXURY

Maybe you can't find a fragrance you love. Maybe you're the sort of person who has their clothes made to measure, and likes everything you do to be touched by individuality. Maybe you're a connoisseur of the finest things in life, on a lifelong quest for the rare, the precious, the unavailable. Maybe you're an oligarch. (Or an oligarch's wife, or his mistress.) There may be many different reasons why an individual turns to a perfumer to commission a bespoke fragrance, with the potential to become their true 'signature scent': true haute couture, in scented form…

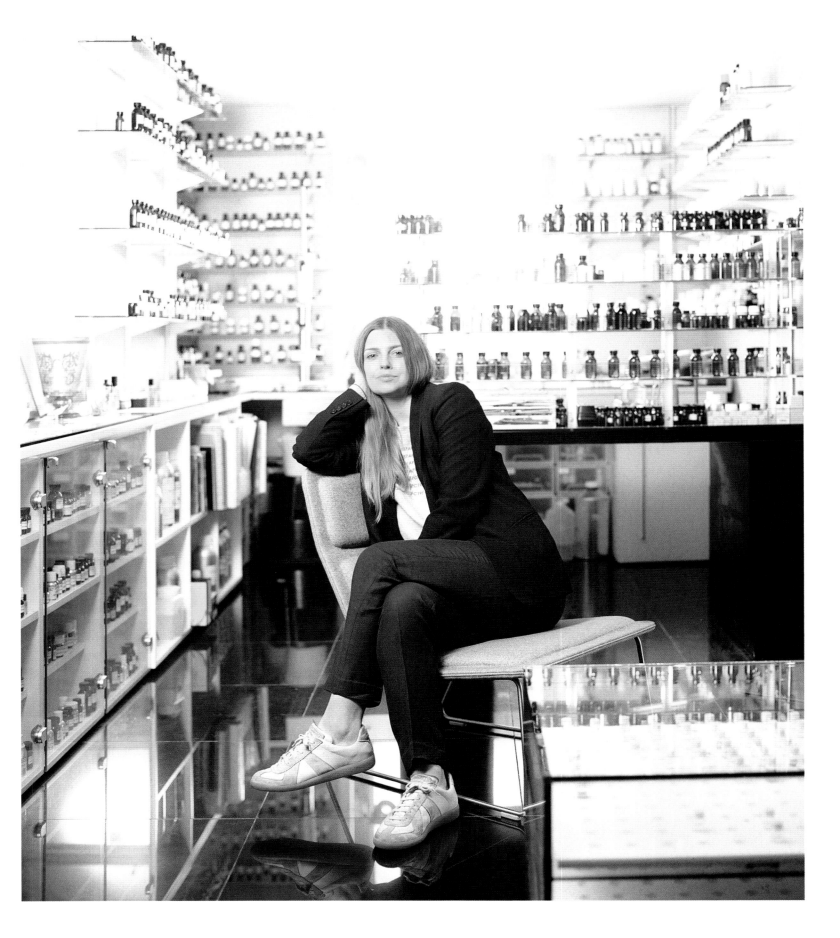

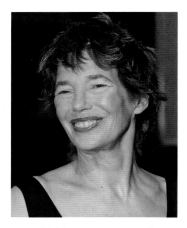

Jane Birkin commissioned Lyn Harris to make L'Air de Rien, which has become a bestseller

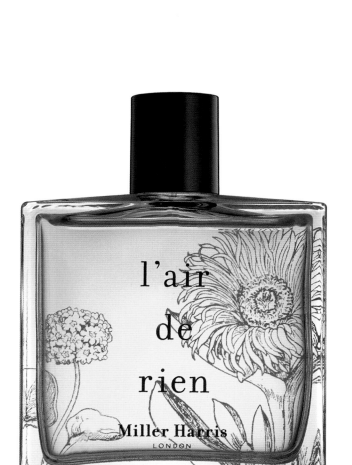

l'air de rien

Miller Harris
LONDON

Commissioning a bespoke perfume isn't cheap. (Although as you'll see at the end of this section, there are some truly accessibly priced options for 'personalising' an existing perfume.) It's one of life's serious luxuries, with a serious price tag to match: Lyn Harris, one of the UK's leading bespoke perfumers, charges from £12,000, often taking more than six months from consultation to pouring the final fragrance into a bottle for a client's delectation.

One of Lyn's celebrated clients was Jane Birkin, who had very clear, individual ideas when she approached Lyn with her perfume notion. Unusually, the fragrance they created ended up being launched commercially as a scent within the Miller Harris portfolio, and L'Air de Rien has become a bestseller. So to understand the process of commissioning a 'personal perfume', we spoke to Lyn at her Notting Hill studio in West London, where clients are invited for that all-important first meeting…

What sort of people come to you for a fragrance?
'Everyone from "the person who has everything" to men who, for instance, have their leather-goods handmade at Hermès, as well as Middle Eastern clients, Far Eastern clients… Sometimes it's a husband wanting to give his wife the ultimate gift. What's interesting is that it often becomes a bit like a "chain letter": I end up creating fragrances for an entire family, or a circle of friends.'

How many bespoke fragrances do you create in a year?
'I can only do four, so I have a waiting list. I need to give it plenty of time, and often these people live overseas, so it's quite a lengthy procedure…'

What does a consultation entail?
'The session can be anything from three to six hours. I start by asking an individual what they already wear, fragrance-wise, and I get their whole timeline: what their mother, their grandmother, their first love wore… It's a bit like psychotherapy, actually: people sometimes turn round and say, "Gosh, I just told you my whole life history!". But it works best when I can really get to know someone in this way; sometimes, if the session's been bought for someone as a present, I get a sense they're feeling "Why am I here?" So my challenge is to break down any resistance. It almost always ends up being hugely enjoyable for both of us.

Do they get to smell things at the session?
'Absolutely, it's a key part of what we do. Right from the word "go" we're smelling materials and they tell me what they like and dislike; I introduce them to the different fragrance families and sub-families, the green notes, the oceanic notes, and so it goes on – dozens and dozens of different things, with me noting down very carefully what pushes someone's buttons.

'I take clients through the natural materials, and also some of the newer materials, and then we work up to some of the jewels of perfumery: the jasmines and roses, etc. They're often surprised at that point, because the raw materials don't smell anything like you'd think, if you're only used to smelling finished perfumes; jasmine can be very medicinal, for instance, yet will become beautifully rich and floral in a finished perfume. Frequent refreshment is often required, in the form of tea, cake and lunch! It's pretty intense. I've had someone faint on me! I had to take him into the garden for a breath of fresh air, but happily, he was fine.'

What happens next?
'By the end of a session, I have three very clear and distinct routes I can go down with the bespoke perfume, and I work on three separate trials, which I present to the client a few months later. Very occasionally, that person loves them all, and I end up making three separate fragrances for them. (In which case, they are charged half the usual fee for the other two fragrances.) But it's never happened that the client's told me: "You've got it all wrong." Never, in 20 years of doing this…

'Often I end up making a candle with the fragrance, so the client can scent his or her home and have that fragrance become even more of a 'signature', inextricably linked with them – in one case, the client liked the candle so much that I ended up making 100 of them as going-home gifts from a party she gave. And clients often ask for body products to be blended with their fragrance, so they can layer the body oil, the body cream – and often they'll ask for five, one for each of their homes.'

What do you love about your bespoke work?
'It's a hugely creative element in what I do. I love the fact that I'm working with money-no-object materials, some of which may be available to me in very small quantities: roses, iris, jasmine, from Grasse and elsewhere, which are often very rare, and which I couldn't incorporate into a fragrance in my own line – costs aside – because I couldn't get my hands on enough of them.

'This creativity feeds into what I do within my own Miller Harris line, too – and not only through projects like Jane Birkin's becoming part of the collection. I'll have ideas, working with my bespoke clients, which lead me down a new path with my next fragrance creation, perhaps opening my eyes to a style I haven't used for a while, or reintroducing me to an ingredient that is a bit of a 'lost love'. I enjoy it all the more because when I told my suppliers in France I was going to be offering bespoke fragrance, they told me I was crazy: "You don't want to be dealing with real people, like that…!" But it's become the most stimulating, exciting dimension of my work.'

Frequent refreshment is often required, in the form of tea, cake and lunch! It's pretty intense. I've had someone faint on me! I had to take him into the garden for a breath of fresh air, but happily, he was fine

Something for (almost) everyone

Did you know that Aveda offers a 'Personal Blend Service', which takes you on a sensory journey to find the scent that will restore your balance, awaken you, soothe you – it's your call, basically. (The 'palette' of ingredients is restricted to naturals; you won't end up with something as complex as a mainstream scent, but it should help you achieve a bit more balance in a c-r-a-z-y world. After you've explored the different key aromas – from bergamot to rose – they're available to you as a Pure-Fume, or for bath and body with Aqua Therapy Salts, Hydrating Lotion or Body Cleanser. Compared to the true bespoke perfumers, it's a steal.

Tailor-made for you

Lyn Harris is one of many gifted perfumers offering a bespoke service, globally. Here's where you might start, in your quest for this ultimate luxury…

Thierry Wasser at Guerlain (Paris) Thierry takes on just a handful of bespoke clients a year for this most exclusive of opportunities: having a fragrance created by the man who's at the creative helm of one of the world's most celebrated fragrance houses.
www.guerlain.com

Roja Dove (London) With his encyclopaedic knowledge of fragrances (and their history), Roja Dove has worked with many private clients to create personal perfumes, a process which costs 'at least' £20,000, and takes many months. He's also created some stunning one-off fragrances for special events, such as the Diaghilev exhibition at London's Victoria & Albert Museum, and a perfume authentic to the time of the Great Fire of London, which could be sniffed, enticingly, though a tiny grille in the wall at an exhibition of The Cheapside Hoard at the Museum of London.
www.rojadove.com

Ormonde Jayne (London) Linda Pilkington (the woman behind Ormonde Jayne) has several jewel-like perfume boutiques in London, but also a thriving private clientele. Although she's not a fully-fledged perfumer, Linda works closely with gifted professionals and often consults with private clients to create the perfume of their dreams and their fantasies.
www.ormondejayne.com

Floris (London) Floris has been creating bespoke perfumes for a long list of celebrated clients since 1730, including countless crowned heads of Europe. In addition to creating bespoke perfumes for individual clients (price £4,500), Floris offers a really surprisingly accessibly-priced 'Fragrance Customisation' consultation: a 90-minute session that ends with the perfumer adding a tailor-made blend of ingredients to personalise one of Floris's existing Fine Fragrance or Private Collection scents.
www.florislondon.com

Anastasia Brozler (London) Globe-trotting Anastasia's 'day job' is working with brands such as Illuminum and Union Fragrance. Her private clients are invited for their consultation into the most stunning offices imaginable (a Georgian building in St. James's). 'I've had clients come in with beautiful antique Hermès handbags wanting to recreate that distinctive

smell of leather, a kind of 1930s chypre. Others drive in with their little Triumph Spitfires and say, "I love the smell of this car leather and crude oil, and I'd like to capture it, combined with my Wellington boots and Barbour jacket, in time for Goodwood." I've been on my hands and knees sniffing exhaust pipes before!'
www.scentlondon.co.uk

Lorenzo Villoresi (Florence) Florentine perfumer Lorenzo Villoresi first studied psychology and philosophy; his travels in North Africa and the Middle East inspired an interest in spices and other fragrant materials, and eventually be began his perfumery career making fragrances for friends. He has his own line of Lorenzo Villoresi perfumes, but also creates bespoke perfumes for an elite clientele.
www.lorenzovilloresi.it

Sarah Horowitz (California) Sarah has been creating custom fragrances since the 1980s, originally toting her fragrance organ (with its 100 oils) around the beaches of Malibu and Los Angeles, conducting 'Fragrance Journeys' and designing custom fragrances for women. A face-to-face consultation is around $1,000 (around £600), though she also offers an interesting 'Online Fragrance Journey' from which three custom formulas (in pure oil) will be created and can be used to create an eau de parfum, shower gel, body lotion, massage oil, etc.
www.sarahhorowitz.com

Mandy Aftel (California) Mandy Aftel (as you can read on pages 70–71) is the world's leading creator of bespoke natural perfumery – but more than that, she was named by Forbes as one of the top seven bespoke perfumers in the world, full-stop – although working only with 100 per cent natural essences and aromas. (Mandy also offers entrancing perfume classes and workshops at her Berkeley studio.)
www.aftelier.com

NB There are many restrictions on shipping fragrance internationally.

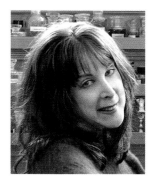

I completely love my materials and I spend a lot of time and a complete fortune sourcing them and then turning them into artisanal fragrances

Mandy Aftel

TIP

Use fragrance to revive lacklustre hair

Our friend Roja Dove advises applying perfume to your hairbrush and sweeping it through your hair. 'It will shine and smell divine.'

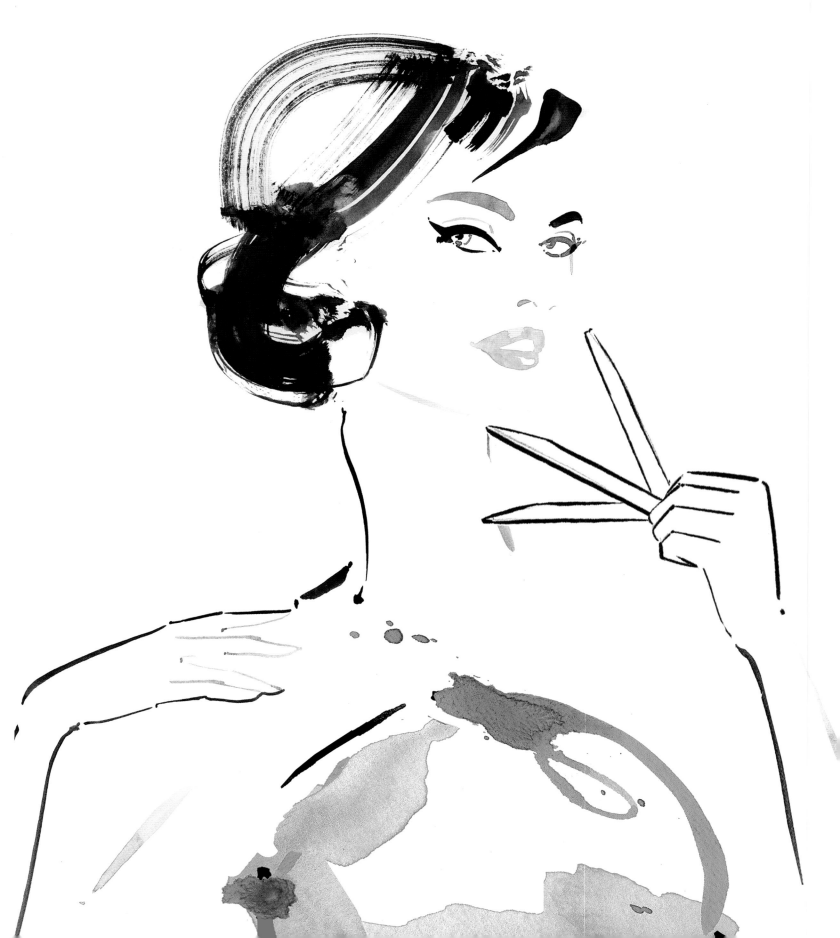

TOP 100 *perfumes* TO TRY *before* YOU DIE

What shaped our selection of these fragrances? In most cases, they're landmark launches of one kind or another *(rather than just a 'me-too')*. Some are pure and simply the most famous fragrances in the world. Others? Well, we simply love them ourselves. There are other beautiful scents out there, for sure – but we think that these are all worth discovering *(and making up your own mind about)* in a lifetime…

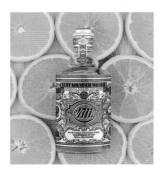

1 4711

Family: Fresh
Launched: 1792
Creator: Wilhelm Meulhens

We wonder: how many fragrances created today will we still be splashing all over in 200 years' time? The answer: a handful, probably (if that). How remarkable, then, that 4711 is pretty much as loved today as it ever was. There's a reason for that: this quintessential eau de Cologne – created in, yes, Cologne – is as refreshing, summery, light and wearable now as it was in 1792, when 4711 debuted. Zestily citrus-heavy, it opens with almost tinglingly uplifting notes of bergamot, orange, neroli – and lemons so juicy they almost squirt you straight in the eye. As the citrus softens, the aromatic heart makes itself known: lavender and rosemary are obvious. (Think: stepping through a gate into an apothecary's garden on a cool evening, with surprisingly powdery roses pulsing their sweetness softly from a sun-warmed wall.) There's a slightly now-you-smell-me-now-you-don't aspect to this entirely unisex scent with faint touches of musk and vetiver in the base.

2 Acqua di Parma Iris Nobile
(eau de parfum)

Family: Chypre
Launched: 2007
Creator: Françoise Caron

Some scents smell similar in different concentrations – but there's a big difference between the luminously light eau de toilette version of this exquisite iris fragrance and the altogether richer, deeper, sexier eau de parfum – which is what we have on our wrists as we write this. Iris Nobile is a truly sensational creation, not at all old-fashioned but with enough 'retro' feel to delight lovers of traditional florals – voluptuous and sexy, but not overpowering. Fragrance notoriously has its own 'fashion moments', and iris was an ingredient du jour for a few years. Few iris scents, though (with the exception of Prada's, and Chanel's divine 28 La Pausa), showcase the sweet, buttery-suede sensuality of this precious, pricy ingredient better than this warm, complex creation by perfumer Françoise Caron (also recipient of the Order of Arts and Literature, a prestigious French cultural award). Notes of bergamot, tangerine, iris, orange blossom, peach and ylang ylang melt into one another, sinking softly into a fantastically long-lasting base of vanilla, patchouli, oakmoss and amber, which pulse gently on the skin. It's like being warmed – by the sun, or an open fire – while the scent from a massive floral arrangement wafts over you.

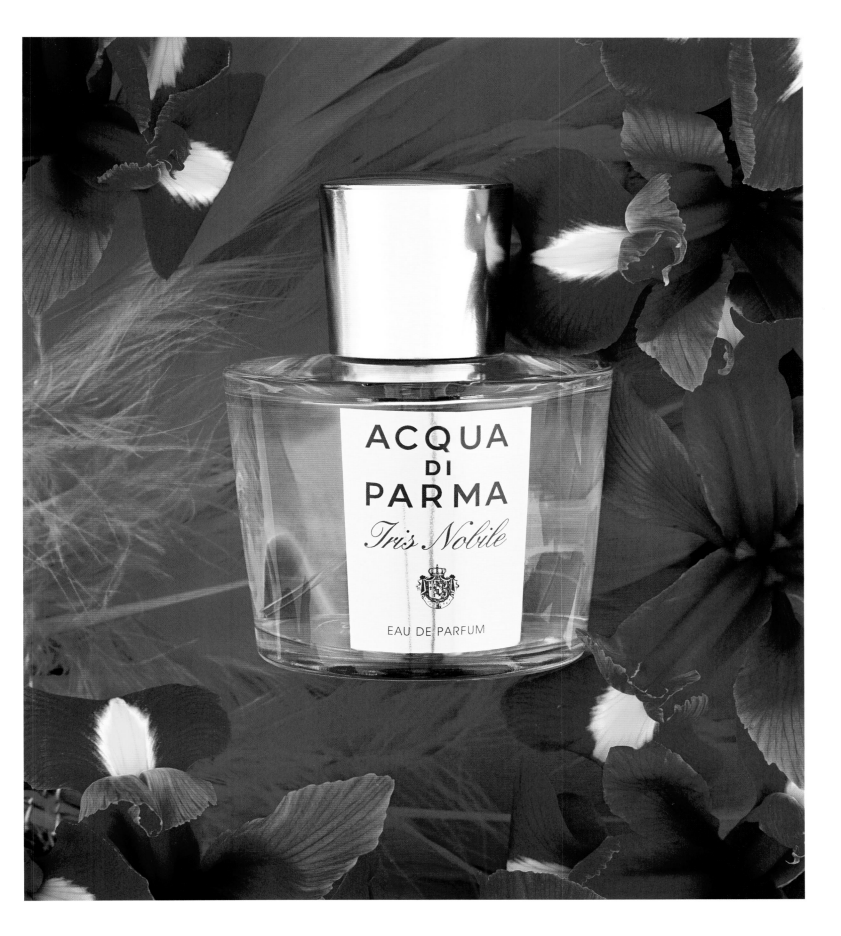

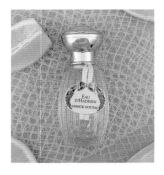

3 Agent Provocateur

Family: Chypre **Launched:** 2000 **Creator:** Christian Provenzano

You just know from the knicker-pink opaque egg-shaped flacon that Agent Provocateur – the debut scent from the saucy lingerie brand – is going to break some rules. And it does: classically 'sexy' scents traditionally fall into the Oriental family, but perfumer Christian Provenzano went down the so-so-sophisticated chypre route with this. There's not much 'striptease' to Agent Provocateur, in terms of getting to know you via the top notes: this beauty's naked lustiness is almost instantly revealed. There's a ton of rose at Agent Provocateur's heart – but not your auntie's rose; this is a raunchy rose. (We love how one perfumista described it on www.basenotes.com: 'This rose has been up all night, smoking and drinking before staggering home as the sun comes up, loving every moment and looking forward to the next time'.) On the skin, it gets more and more sensual, rich in patchouli and leather, smouldering alongside smoky amber, musk and oakmoss. Not one for the office, we advise – but if you've seduction in mind…? Slip into your very best underwear, spritz liberally – and maybe you'll still be able to make out subtle, lingeringly sensual traces on your skin when you're making espresso for two next morning.

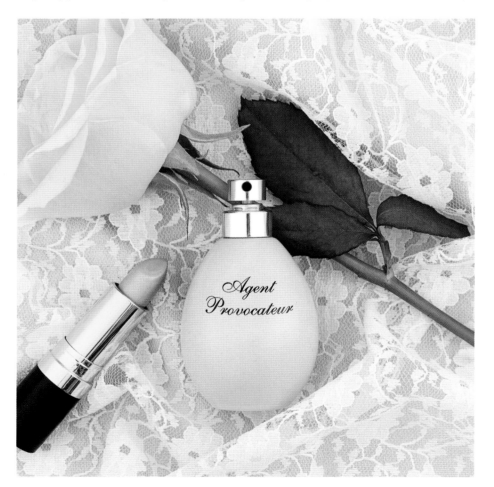

4 Annick Goutal Eau d'Hadrien

Family: Fresh
Launched: 1981
Creators: Annick Goutal and Francis Camail

This sherbet lemon-y, airy confection set perfumer Annick Goutal on the path to stardom. Technically, Eau d'Hadrien is a 'shared' scent, thanks to its luminous freshness – which works equally well on male and female skins. At the get-go, there's a ton of citrus – grapefruit, Sicilian lemon, citron, mandarin orange. Its 'luminous' quality, meanwhile, is down to aldehydes: the same synthetic ingredients that 'power' Chanel No. 5, making it almost burst fizzily from the bottle. The short-lived citrus notes don't hang around – but that's not the end of things: there are some herbal notes, and a touch of pencil-case cypress. For softness, a trace of ylang ylang, too – but there's nothing to tip this unisex classic into the realms of girliness. If it's a love affair with citrus you're after, Eau d'Hadrien is as simple and uncomplicated as it gets. Bottom line: this has a washing-on-the-line, breezy outdoorsiness – and if you love stepping out of a shower and putting on a clean white shirt, it's for you. Unlike the more sophisticated, complex Orientals and florals, the whole 'fresh' family of scents is relatively fleeting on the skin. But re-spritzing this uplifting, energising creation is part of the joy.

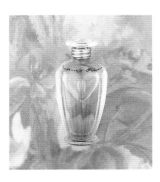

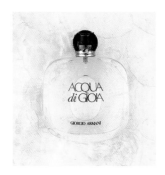

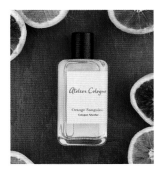

5 Antonia's Flowers

Family: Floral
Launched: 1984
Creator: Bernard Chant

Nobody has ever really captured the smell of walking into a florist's shop the way Antonia Bellanca did, with this. Her Long Island florist's became a Mecca for the Hamptons elite, and its success inspired Antonia to work with a perfumer to bottle that slightly mossy, wet, ferny, lush aroma. One note stands head and shoulders above every other, though: the freesia, which kicks in straight after the high-octane rush you get when you first unstopper the pretty pale pink juice. We're not sure why this so-pretty note isn't more widely used (or recreated), but freesia is certainly abundant here, faithfully recapturing the moment you bury your nose in a bunch of these flowers. We get whispers of other florals, too – violet in particular, honeysuckle, maybe an aromatic lavender note (plus a hint of refreshing Earl Grey tea) – but what's amazing about Antonia's Flowers is its absolute dewiness. It never goes powdery, but stays crisp and green throughout. If you love buying flowers, or want something that really does cram spring into a bottle, Antonia's Flowers is it. And trust us: whenever you wear it, people will ask what scent you've got on; it quite simply smells like nothing else.

6 Armani Acqua di Gioia *(eau de parfum)*

Family: Fresh
Launched: 2010
Creators: Loc Dong, Anne Flipo and Dominique Ropion

Sometimes when you want to cool yourself down with a fresh fragrance, you'll reach for a good old eau de Cologne. Other times, you'll want something that brings down your temperature but speaks of cool sea breezes – and this fresh-scented Armani creation delivers: the fragrant equivalent of a long, chilled glass of cucumber-flavoured water, with its thirst-slaking power. Almost everything about this is sheer and transparent: at first, a slightly tart lemonade-fruitiness, with juicier fruit undertones of grapefruit and (we sense) pineapple. In the equally transparent heart, you'll encounter swags of lemon blossom and aromatic crushed mint, lots of greenness, with some jasmine twining through, and a touch of pepper. For those first two phases, there's a definite aquatic quality to Acqua di Gioia. But as it warms on the skin, the fragrance's complexity drifts in: woody cedar and labdanum (from the Mediterranean 'rock rose') are mellowed by the sweetness of a 'brown sugar accord', which adds a merest hint of 'edible' gourmand softness to the base. Fresh and so, so summery, we just can't imagine wearing this in winter.

7 Atelier Cologne Orange Sanguine

Family: Fresh
Launched: 2010
Creator: Ralph Schwieger

Who doesn't love that invigorating moment when you plunge your fingers into orange peel, and experience a zingy burst of juice…? Atelier Cologne's fresh and elegant Orange Sanguine almost magically captures that – one of the first fragrances in their collection of 'Colognes-plus', designed to have much longer staying power than most. (Read more about AC's philosophy on page 85.) 'Orange Sanguine' translates as blood orange, and this is citrus a gogo, (almost) with the bitterness of peel in the top notes offsetting the sweet juiciness of the orange itself. After that sun-drenched opening, the heart of the fragrance morphs into something more cool and 'green': notes of geranium and a low-key jasmine, with a touch of black pepper, gradually warming up as the tonka bean, amber woods and sandalwood creep in. Orange Sanguine won the 'Experts Award' in the French FiFi (Fragrance Foundation) Awards in 2012, one of the highest accolades the industry can bestow – and deservedly so. If you don't yet know Atelier Cologne, find a perfumery which showcases their so-interesting work – and enjoy an orange 'hit' from this, which we swear almost delivers a jolt of vitamin C.

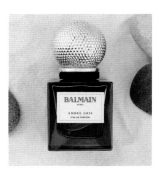

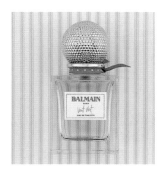

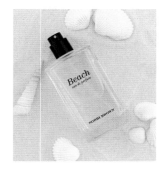

8 Balmain Ambre Gris

Family: Oriental
Launched: 2008
Creator: Guillaume Flavigny

Ambergris is one of perfume's sacred and mysterious ingredients – impossible to plan for: it simply washes up on the shore – produced, um, by a whale's digestive system... How anything so unglamorous can smell so hauntingly seductive is mind-boggling, but it does. (If you ever get the chance to smell genuine ambergris, it's unforgettably wonderful.) And even though this creation from the newly revived Balmain couture house uses a synthetic representation of ambergris, it's enough to give a sense of how beguiling the coveted real ingredient is. Blink and you'll miss the pink berries and sage that open this scent, before its fabulous soft, spicy heart opens up: cinnamon, resinous myrrh, little trails of incense – we get black pepper, too. Ambre Gris isn't 'in your face' like many Orientals, but it still lasts and lasts on the skin: a fabulous fog of amber and smoke, white musk and benzoin, a vanilla-esque ingredient that makes this almost good-enough-to-eat. Bottom line: Ambre Gris is as cocooning as a cashmere shawl, as comforting as a cup of cocoa – but oh, a lot sexier than both. (We love the Deco-style cap and the chic grey glass, too – straight out of *The Great Gatsby*.)

9 Balmain Vent Vert

Family: Floral
Launched: 1945
Creator: Germaine Cellier

'Green wind' isn't much of a name for a fragrance; 'Vent Vert' (the French original) is somehow so much more evocative, conjuring up the green 'gusts' that have been captured in this bottle. The newly-reworked Vent Vert isn't, actually, nearly as unmistakably green as the original – but you still get hints of what creator Germaine Cellier, one of the few female perfumers working at that time, was after: the freshness of cut grass, the cool of the shade under an evergreen, with a slight (we'd say almost acrid) dryness, too, from labdanum, galbanum, as well as aromatic basil.(Cellier was quite a woman: her other 'cult' creations include the iconic tuberose Fracas and Bandit, for Robert Piguet, as well as Jolie Madame for Balmain. Hats off, Germaine.) Floral notes have now been revved up to make Vent Vert more alluring to the modern perfume-wearer; allegedly the composition has been edited down from 1,100 ingredients to just 30, to include violet, freesia, hyacinth, ylang ylang, lily of the valley, iris and neroli. It is crisp, fresh, a little bit shyer than it was – but we still love it, even if the lovely powdery finish of old isn't so much in evidence.

10 Bobbi Brown Beach

Family: Floral
Launched: 2002
Creator: Unattributed

Summertime, and the living is easy... Well, it certainly is with this, Bobbi Brown's bestselling fragrance. This smells of youth and summer, carefree sunny days that go on forever: skin slathered in suntan lotion, sand sticking to it, flip-flops and shorts, Beach Boys blasting out from a speaker somewhere... Mostly, that completely free-as-a-bird feeling becomes all too rare as responsibilities settle into our lives, but can be magically evoked with a spritz of this. It's jasmine and neroli, wafted at you on a breeze of marine notes and with an extraordinary saltiness that almost makes you want to lick your skin. Do women want to smell like suntan lotion? Well, yes, sometimes we do. And if you want to close your eyes and be on vacation in a microsecond, there's nothing that'll get you there quicker. The make-up artist's scent line deserves to have as high a profile as her like-you-but-prettier make-up, so it is worth exploring when next you're stocking up on taupe eyeshadow. Our absolute favourite is Bed: the longest lasting orange blossom ever, in the form of a perfume oil. Alas, it comes and goes as an occasionally revived limited edition – so we grab it when we can.

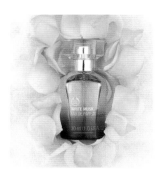

11 The Body Shop White Musk

Family: Floriental
Launched: 1981
Creator: Unattributed

Ah, White Musk… For decades, Britain's teenage girls smelled of nothing else. (And plenty of grown-up, super-sophisticated women we know have never moved on from it.) What's extraordinary, to us, is that aside from Chanel No. 5 we can't think of a fragrance that evokes such a misty-eyed nostalgia among wearers; one breath and the decades melt away. But who could have guessed, when The Body Shop unveiled this at the start of the 1980s, that it would go on to become an (affordable) perfume 'icon', remaining one of their bestsellers today…? The lingering base notes in White Musk, meanwhile, are innocent 'clean musks' rather than a down-and-dirty muskiness: sweet and fluffy cloud-y, with pretty, powdery floral notes that dry down to a gentle vanilla cosiness on the skin. Smelling it again years after we left school locker rooms behind, we think it truly deserves its place in women's hearts. And while you're checking it out, do explore the White Musk Perfume Oil, which is darker and more smouldering, complex with notes of lily, ylang ylang, jasmine and rose – perhaps a new way to experience and enjoy White Musk, if you fancy a trip down memory lane?

12 Bottega Veneta Eau de Parfum

Family: Chypre **Launched:** 2011 **Creator:** Michael Almairac

We absolutely love it when a perfume house avoids taking the 'safe route' when creating their debut scent and we love that Bottega Veneta, the ultra-luxe Venetian leather goods brand, opted to create a glorious modern chypre to put itself on the perfume map. This really is one for leather-lovers: even though leather isn't even mentioned in the ingredients pyramid, Bottega Veneta has a buttery-soft, touch-me suede sensuality (helped along by a heavy dose of iris and violet). It also features the classic chypre 'pillars' of bergamot in the top and oakmoss and patchouli in the base, but in between swirls a seriously elegant, velvety Venetian fog of jasmine, together with little whispers of pink pepper and ripe fruit: we get apricot and plum, plus musk and vanilla. We agree with a couple of bloggers who've observed that there's a sort of 'salty tang' to Bottega Veneta, too, like the distant smell of the sea that you get inland. (It's there because, according to nose Michel Almairac, 'ports smell of leather'.) With its Murano glass bottle (check out the Bottega Veneta 'woven' base) and a teeny sliver of leather round the neck, the whole package feels (and smells) seriously luxurious.

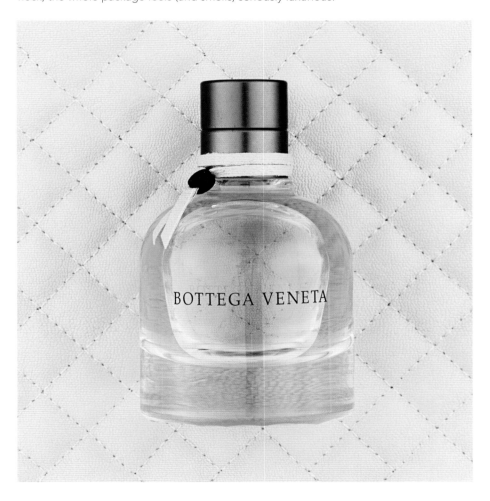

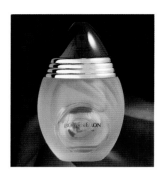

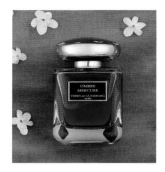

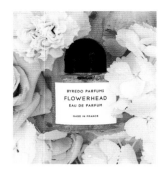

13 Boucheron Boucheron

Family: Floral
Launched: 1989
Creators: Francis Deleamont and Jean-Pierre Bethouart

We love fragrance's mood-shifting power – and should you find yourself in a slump at the end of a hard day, with a glamorous evening stretching ahead of you and absolutely no will to slip into a Little Black Dress, a spritz of this opulent floral from the ring-inspired flacon on to your pulse-points should put you in the mood to celebrate faster than you can say 'Moët & Chandon'. This seductive debut scent from Paris's jewellery house is a gem itself: complex, intriguing and dressed-up, from first dab or spritz through to the last trace that lingers on your velvet jacket when you finally put it back on the hanger. (Or fling it over the back of a chair, if the evening's lived up to its promise…) Basil and pelargonium open, before feminine white flowers unfurl their petals: ylang ylang, orange blossom, tuberose, jasmine. After a while, the base notes trumpet their presence: woods and vanilla, oakmoss and tonka bean, ambergris, musk and civet (these 'animalic' notes now synthetic, as across most of the fragrance industry today). Even the eau de parfum is long-lasting on the skin, and fairly heavy in nature – which is why it's just so party-perfect.

14 By Terry Ombre Mercure

Family: Floral **Launched:** 2012
Creators: Jacques Fleury, Arthur Le Tourneur d'Ison, Karine Vinchon and Sidonie Lancesseur

You may perhaps know Terry de Gunzburg as a make-up artist with her own upscale signature range. Though fairly recently launched, the perfectionist Terry worked on her debut collection of five scents for 14 – yes, 14 – years. And it shows. Reluctantly forced to single out one from the collection, it had to be the velvety, rich Ombre Mercure, which has all the magic of a vintage scent. As Terry says, 'I wanted to reconnect with perfumes from the beginning of the last century, like those of Guerlain and Robert Piguet – they were extravagant experiences. That's not to say mine are dusty old fragrances. They're contemporary – clean but not watery, opulent but not heavy'. Oodles of soft, rounded violet and iris certainly offer Guerlainesque echoes here, giving a velvetiness that's further enhanced by lots of honeyed vanilla. Drifts of rose, jasmine, patchouli and ylang ylang just add to the deliciousness – we can't do better than to quote Terry on this: 'Intense, powerful and purring on the skin just like a feline'.

15 Byredo Flowerhead

Family: Floral
Launched: 2014
Creators: Olivia Giacobetti and Jérôme Epinette

It took Swedish perfume brand Byredo's Ben Gorham six years, we're told, to complete Flowerhead (in collaboration with the perfumers named above) – but it was sure worth the wait. The inspiration was the memory of a cousin's wedding in Jaipur, India, where garlands of fresh blooms are central to the ceremony, even woven into the bride's hair – giving rise to the name, 'Flowerhead'. This is a massive bouquet of flowers, itself: a classic floral, crammed full of notes like rose, tuberose and jasmine, but with a lightness of touch that ensures it's not in the least 'vintage'. Flowerhead opens with a burst of dew-drenched citrus and tart berries (lemon, green notes, angelica seeds, lingonberry), before the flowers appear in a procession. (Jasmine's the bride, tuberose and rose are the maids-of-honour.) It stays spring-like and fresh throughout, despite the notes of woods and musks which gradually emerge – and almost everyone we know who's smelled this has fallen in love. In fact one young woman – who we gave our bottle to – simply declared, 'I used to get dressed and apply my perfume. Now I stand there and spray this all over, and then put my clothes on.' What greater endorsement?

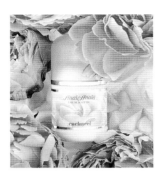

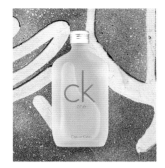

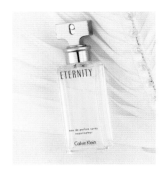

16 Cacharel Anaïs Anaïs

Family: Floral
Launched: 1978
Creators: Paul Leger, Raymond Chaillan, Roger Pellegrino and Robert Gonnon

For a decade or two it seemed as if the whole of Europe smelled of this blockbuster: Anaïs Anaïs was the first scent for droves of young women who still feel nostalgic at a whiff of its soft white floral powderiness. There's a fleeting leafy green herbaceous moment at the start, but really this is delicately flower-powered: lily, lily of the valley, rose, ylang ylang, tuberose, carnation, melting sweetly into one another. In some hands, those blooms can be projected as opulent, extravagant, voluptuous – but this is all innocence and tenderness, see-through and floaty, echoed in the soft-focus 1920s-style advertising by photographer Sarah Moon. The base notes are subtle: oakmoss, sandalwood, cedarwood and amber; after a while, there's a sort of powered wood aspect and an almost chypre sophistication. It's way more refined than the bubblegummy florals most 16-year-olds seem to fall for – and we think it could work at any age. No doubt there are some very grown-up fans who've never budged from this scent – and smelling it again, we find ourselves thinking: maybe they're on to something.

17 Calvin Klein ck one

Family: Fresh
Launched: 1994
Creators: Alberto Morillas and Harry Fremont

ck one kicked off a trend for 'shared' scents when it debuted – and suddenly, they weren't just unisex, but sexy, too. Ann Gottlieb, creative director of many of Calvin Klein's fragrances, describes this as 'jumping in the air, just showered after a warm day'. It was a massive instant success, notching up an unprecedented $5 million in business in the first ten days alone and went on to become so popular that it felt like you could smell it everywhere: so-fresh gusts of bergamot, lemon, mandarin, with hedione (a jasmine-derived ingredient) in the heart, touches of tropical fruit (pineapple, papaya), alongside violet, rose and tiny sprinklings of nutmeg and cardamom spice. It's definitely clean, clean, clean: for a while, this type of uncomplicated fresh scent dominated – and ck one spawned a thousand copies, skewing the whole mood of perfumery towards purity and cleanliness, rather than voluptuous sex and seduction. Something else marked it out: the utilitarian-looking bottle with a metal screw top (albeit designed by one of the greatest graphic designers ever, Fabien Baron). But it has stood the test: ck one now looks completely timeless. And smells it, too.

18 Calvin Klein Eternity

Family: Floral
Launched: 1988
Creator: Sophia Grojsman

We've a hunch: this enduring blockbuster is probably the fragrance that has been worn for more weddings than any other in history. (What's in a name? Everything, when it comes to Eternity.) There's a lovely story behind it: the scent was inspired by the eternity ring that King Edward VIII gave to Wallis Simpson – and which fashion designer Calvin Klein later bought at auction for his then wife, photographer Kelly Proctor. Aptly, it's a bouquet-in-a-bottle, too – spicy hints of carnation, before the rampant roses swirl in. Despite touches of vanilla-y heliotrope, it's not over-sweet: lily of the valley and other green notes give Eternity its sophistication. It's very bride-appropriate: you don't want anything too over-the-top sexy for a wedding – and this is sensual without being voluptuous. We'd say it almost has a virginal 'cleanness': a tad soapy (in an expensive soap way. And we love a bar of expensive soap.) In the base are synthetic musks, known for not budging from the skin for days – so in other words: if you did wear it for a wedding, your new husband would be able to smell your neck and get hints of Eternity, the-morning-after-the-hopefully-memorable-night-before.

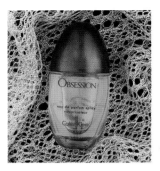

19 Calvin Klein Obsession

Family: Oriental
Launched: 1985
Creator: Jean Guichard

It's hard to imagine now how hot under the collar people got about Obsession's advertising: a dimly-lit tangle of perfect naked bodies, promoting an unashamedly erotic fragrance. Calvin Klein's debut scent, Obsession is unusually powerful, even for an Oriental: a light-the-blue-touch-paper-and-retire sort of fragrance, designed to set off major fireworks. The brief from creative director Ann Gottleib was 'sensuality with a touch of raunch' and 'classy with a touch of trash'. There are top notes (mandarin, bergamot) and heart notes (ylang ylang, orange flower), for sure but it sprints right to the base, almost barely pausing in the top and heart. The way it then flaunts the base notes is positively carnal: frankincense, amber, civet, oakmoss, musk, vetiver, amber – and lots and lots of vanilla. Obsession was specifically formulated to last all night and into the morning – and truly, it does. (NB Over the years, there's been some reformulation of Obsession – but quite a few fans find it more wearable.) The bottle of cognac-coloured juice is pebble-smooth and pretty sensual in its own right – but please: don't wear this to the office, unless you've got a co-worker firmly in your seductive sights.

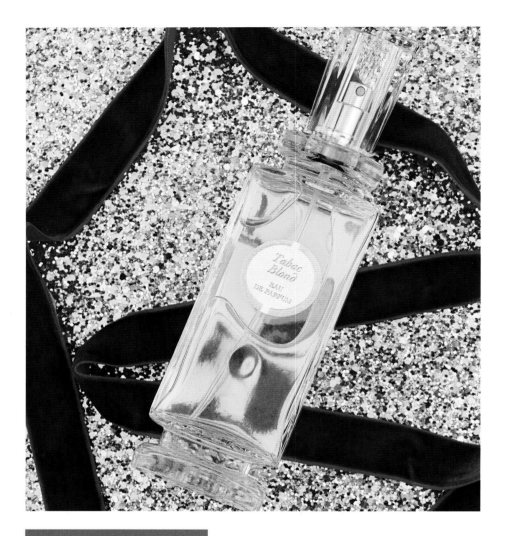

20 Caron Tabac Blond

Family: Chypre **Launched:** 1919 **Creator:** Ernest Daltroff

Created just after the First World War ended by the House of Caron's founder, Ernest Daltroff, Tabac Blond is actually quintessentially 1920s: a fragrance for a time when women were discovering their independence. It's charlestons and over-made-up silent movie stars and Lucky Strike cigarettes and illegal hooch: daringly naughty, especially for that time in history – but delicious with it. Smell it on a blotter and you may get a hit of nose-tinglingly, powdery, clove-spicy carnation. But apply to the skin and Tabac Blond becomes infinitely more interesting. You won't get much from the 'heart' of this vintage creation; the base notes rush straight into the party: a fug of mysterious incense, luxurious leatheriness, a pulsing amber warmth. Add to that a sort of crème brûlée sweetness, a stable-ful of leather and enough patchouli to satisfy anyone's inner hippie – though perhaps not as much tobacco as the name implies. (Officially, the notes also include linden, vetiver, cedar, ambergris and musk.) Tabac Blond's sillage (or its 'lasting' quality) can be measured almost in days, and this isn't one for work, either.

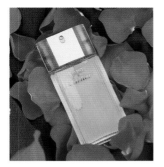

21 Cartier La Panthère

Family: Chypre **Launched:** 2014 **Creator:** Mathilde Laurent

Cartier is one of the few fragrance houses to have their own in-house 'nose', the off-the-scale-talented Mathilde Laurent, who was swimming against a tide of fruity-florals when she created this new, super-chic chypre. As Mathilde explained to us at the time of launch, this whole exquisite fragrance family is 'endangered': perfumers are generally scared to use the key chypre ingredient oakmoss (which has been restricted for reasons of sensitivity). So fragrance suppliers don't offer it. So perfumers can't use it… We couldn't be more pleased that Mathilde has done her bit to keep chypre alive with this 'feline floral', with its peachy coloured 'juice'. Lots of sparkling gardenia, teensy touches of fruit – tart rhubarb and strawberry, from an interesting molecule called 'styrallyl acetate' – but it includes animalic notes, too: musk and, yes, plenty of oakmoss. It's super-sexy and very, very sophisticated – and the bottle's one of the most stunning we've seen launched in many a year, with a 'panther' profile, carved into the inside of the glass flacon. This big cat absolutely purrs at you – and if 'feline floral' turns out to be a whole new fragrance family, we're all in for some treats.

22 Cartier Must de Cartier

Family: Oriental
Launched: 1981
Creator: Jean-Jacques Diener

Oriental fragrances are all smoulder and seduction, generally – so the in-your-face green whiff of galbanum (a resin extracted from rock rose) is a surprise here, at first spritz. Must is fresh – but sultry at the same time. And according to fragrance überexpert Michael Edwards, there's a reason for that: as with many fragrances, a 'brief' was put out to different creators, but Cartier was dithering between a fresh fragrance or an Oriental. A young nose at perfume house Givaudan meshed the two together and got the gig. As the bright green 'gust' drifts away, your nose should get a hint of neroli and mandarin before sweeter notes waft softly in: narcissus, hedione (from jasmine) and rose. It's really the musky, ambery base of Must that hooks us: a seductive interplay of vanilla, benzoin resin, sandalwood, opopanax, with animalic civet (a synthetic, nowadays, but very raunchy nonetheless). Le Must was the first fragrance from the house known as 'the jeweller of kings and the king of jewellers'; in the 1970s, they moved into more 'wearable' (and affordable) everyday jewels, watches and lighters – and this. A bit of a gem, we think.

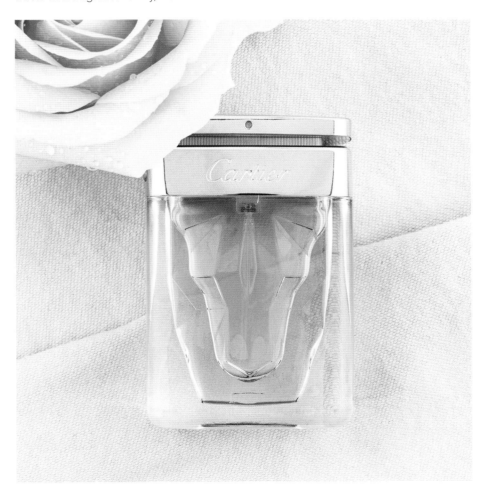

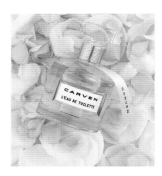

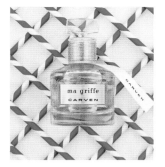

23 Carven Le Parfum

Family: Floral
Launched: 2013
Creator: Francis Kurkdjian

Some fragrances have 'instant classic' written all over them, the minute we first smell them – and this is one. Carven Le Parfum is not something you'd wear to seduce a lover, though: this delicate petal floral is a scent you can get away with wearing to the office without upsetting colleagues, or leaving traces behind you in the lift you took to the 25th floor. (You could even wear it to an interview – and there aren't many perfumes we'd recommend for that.) Definitely more 'personal' and intimate than many of today's in-your-face creations, a rain shower of fresh petals mists over you to start with: pretty, pretty, pretty. Those petals themselves include lots of sweet pea, alongside mandarin blossom, jasmine, neroli and hyacinth. Base notes are subtle, yet still quietly there: soft musks and woods and a whisper of patchouli – but it's all put together with a featherlight touch by Francis Kurkdjian; read more about this 'star' of the fragrance world on page 89. The woman who wears his airy creation, meanwhile, probably sits up straight in her chair, exuding a calm, well-groomed elegance – while managing to keep her crisp white shirt uncrumpled all day long.

24 Carven Ma Griffe

Family: Chypre
Launched: 1946
Creator: Jean Carles

Ma Griffe – which means 'my signature' – had surely one of the coolest launches ever: the brand dropped hundreds of tiny green-and-white parachutes from the skies of Paris, each of which carried a sample of Madame Carven's signature scent. Ma Griffe was recognised as one of the great chypres of its time. Aldehydes add airiness to the short-lived orange blossom and citrus elements, at first sniff. In the heart is a relatively understated bouquet of florals, including ylang ylang, rose, lily of the valley, jasmine, lily, orris root (from iris), oh-so-lightly sweetened with a squirt of peach. There are plenty of 'green' elements, though, which stop this being girly-girly and propel it into the realms of intrigue: clary sage and the Indian spice asfoetida, extracted from a type of giant fennel. The real difference seems to be that today, the sexy base (vetiver, musk, benzoin and styrax) has been lightened up quite a bit, but overall the whole impression is polished, smooth, seamless, with no hard edges. In its somewhat reworked current incarnation, Ma Griffe remains sophisticated and still so wearable – but more intimate, rather than the head-turning, sharp-suited power perfume which scented all of post-war Paris.

25 Chanel Coco

Family: Oriental
Launched: 1984
Creator: Jacques Polge

Coco strode into our lives in the 80s, a time of power-shouldered suits, OTT costume jewellery and take-no-prisoners va-va-voom scents for take-no-prisoners women. A spicy Oriental, Coco swirls with cardamom, cumin, carnation-like clove, cinnamon: resinous and warm and elegantly sexy. In classic Chanel style, Coco is blasted out of the bottle on a surge-tide of aldehydes, delivering mandarin peel, orange and peach – which barely have time to stop and say 'hello' before Coco really starts to sizzle, introducing opulent notes of rose and jasmine, orange blossom and clove buds. Unusually, there's a note from cascarilla, a West Indian shrub with a bark used to flavour liqueur. The base thrums with sandalwood, patchouli, tonka, leather and labdanum, plus a 'secret ingredient', Prunol, which gives a rich, dark, dried-fruit-and-spices depth to Coco, creating an almost chocolatey sensuality. Coco is the absolute perfume equivalent of the Chanel handbag, the double-C earrings: most definitely an accessory, a finishing touch. If you worry about such things, Coco is incredibly economical: a few drops in contact with skin or clothes will cocoon you in their sensual warmth for hours and hours, trailing Oriental loveliness in your wake.

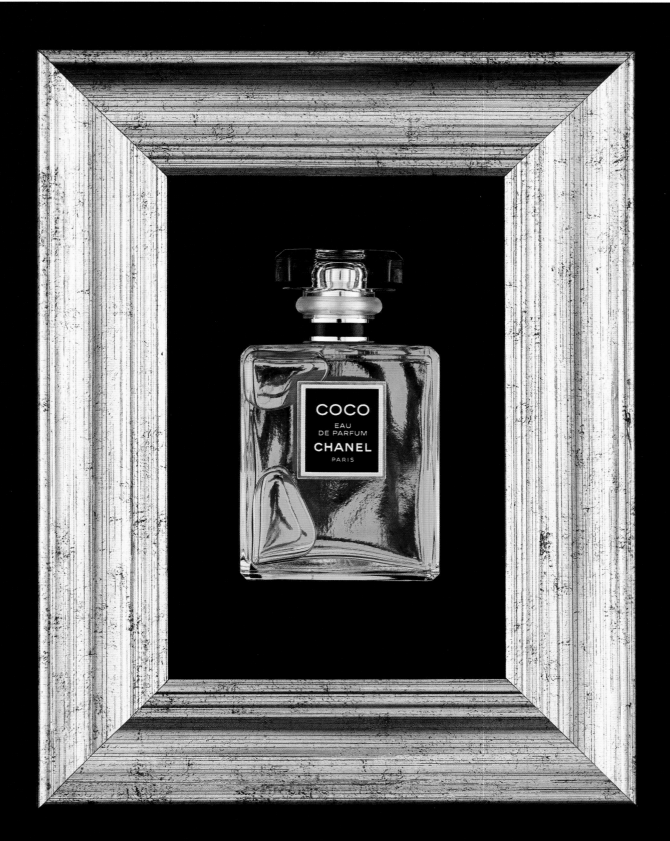

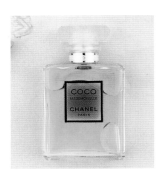

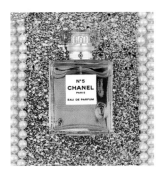

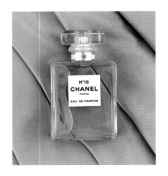

26 Chanel Coco Mademoiselle

Family: Chypre
Launched: 2001
Creator: Jacques Polge

You might not want your daughter to leave the house in Chanel's original Coco (read about this so-sexy Oriental on the previous page) – but you'd be thrilled if she spritzed this behind her ear. Young, airy, pretty-pretty-pretty, this is the perfume equivalent of Karl Lagerfeld designing sneakers for the Chanel label: fun and youthful and fresh. (And hey, if that's how you see yourself, Mademoiselle works at any age.) There's a lot of 'gourmand' to Mademoiselle: edible notes of lychee, fleeting whispers of orange, grapefruit and lemon, all drizzled with vanilla. Rose and jasmine weave in and out in quite a hazy way; what's quite definitely 'there' is patchouli, in generous quantities: a love-it-or-hate-it note, nestling beside musk and vetiver. (We're in the 'adore' camp: patchouli's much more than a 'hippie' note.) A word on 'layering' Mademoiselle: there are some really fabulous body products to complement the different strengths of 'juice': soaps, oils, lotions – answering all sorts of gift problems for what to buy the Mademoiselle-lover. And there are a lot of them about: Mademoiselle is consistently one of the top-selling fragrances in the US, beating even its legendary stablemate, No. 5. Wow.

27 Chanel No. 5

Family: Floral
Launched: 1921
Creator: Ernest Beaux

It's almost impossible to put pen to paper to write about Chanel No. 5 without diving straight into the realms of cliché. It remains a global bestseller, the most recognised fragrance name in the world, getting on for 90 years since Ernest Beaux first slipped with a vial of aldehydes, so the legend goes, and sloshed an overdose into one of the blends he was creating for the very discerning couturier Mademoiselle Gabrielle Chanel. Miss Picky-Picky herself worked through the numbered samples, stopped at No. 5 – and the rest (literally) is fragrance history. It has utterly classic proportions: almost a fizz of effervescent aldehydic top notes jostling for head space with ylang ylang (then softened as the orange blossom emerges), a jasmine and rose heart, sandalwood and vetiver in the base… It is the most soigné fragrance a woman could wish for. As Chanel's in-house perfumer Jacques Polge observes, 'When Mademoiselle Chanel created the fragrance, her idea was that the bottle should be as simple as possible and everything should be in the fragrance.' Despite the challenges of reworking Chanel No. 5 under ever-tighter restrictions on natural ingredients, it remains miraculously unchanged.

28 Chanel No. 19

Family: Floral
Launched: 1971
Creator: Henri Robert

Allegedly, this was Coco Chanel's favourite fragrance. She named it after her birthday (19th August). And initially, she reserved No. 19 for special friends and clients. Worked on by Henri Robert, it was finally launched in 1971, becoming one of the 'signature' scents of that decade and introducing Chanel fragrances to a younger, newly independent generation. It's now a timeless floral-chypre classic, with a cool breeze of the greenest notes blowing through it. (In fact, if you've ever wondered what galbanum smells like – the tart, resinous extract from the cistus, aka rock rose, plant – just spray a touch of No. 19 on your skin.) It tells of grassy meadows and outdoorsiness. The galbanum's dominant, to start with, but then gently wafts off, allowing the floral heart to soften No. 19's greenness: jasmine, roses, orris (iris), narcissus, lily of the valley and ylang ylang. Unlike many contemporary scents, in which what you spritz at the counter is pretty much what you still have on your skin hours later, No. 19 reveals itself very languidly. In the base, with a crisp-white-sheets musk, sandalwood and lots of grounding vetiver. We rediscovered No. 19 for this book – and have fallen right back in love.

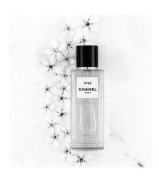

29 Chanel No. 22
(now in Chanel Les Exclusifs collection)

Family: Floral
Launched: 1922
Creator: Ernest Beaux

Everyone, but everyone, knows Chanel's No. 5 – but we think this deserves to be just as famous: it's richer, more complex, utterly exquisite. Named after the year of its launch and created by Ernest Beaux (who created No. 5 itself), this is crystal clear and crisp when you first spray it – lots and lots of aldehydes, which make you feel as if your lungs have been filled with oxygen on a clear summer's day, and add a serious sparkle factor to the neroli and lily of the valley top notes. Then the headier white flowers romp in – tuberose, jasmine, rose, ylang ylang – and hang around for ages. Gradually, the spices, woods (vetiver) and incense emerge – plus a more obvious dash of vanilla than No. 5, giving No. 22 a lingering sensual intensity. (Put it on a teenager and it's the equivalent of a toddler slipping into Mummy's heels.) And we've a hunch: if you're a No. 5 addict and you dabble in No. 22, there's no going back. In addition, we recommend the perfume itself, rather than the lighter versions: a dab on the throat and you're already halfway transported to dinner or the theatre, as if by magic.

30 Clinique Aromatics Elixir
Family: Chypre **Launched:** 1971 **Creator:** Bernard Chant

Aromatics Elixir still smells like nothing else out there: a swirl of spices, exotic flowers, almost camphor-y and even a touch medicinal, at fleeting moments. And if you're not familiar with Aromatics Elixir, we'll bet you've smelled it a hundred times on strangers, without realising. Aromatics Elixir is a chypre, with all the usual chypre elements: bergamot, oakmoss, cistus and patchouli. But there's also carnation and tuberose beating loudly at its heart, alongside vetiver and sandalwood and resiny notes, musk and hints of rose. Some fragrances are the equivalent of stepping into Mummy's shoes (see Chanel No. 22, left) – but for a young woman (we were, when we first wore this), it wasn't just akin to slipping into her heels, but borrowing her fur coat, nicking the car keys and her Balkan Sobranie cigarettes and going for a long, illegal drive! If you're drawn to fruity-florals or sugary gourmands, this might seem like going from daylight into a velvet-curtained, thumping nightclub. But we think it's really worth exploring, not just on a blotter. Because, as your skin warms the spices and those seductive base notes, will you 'get' why Aromatics Elixir is still going strong after more than four decades.

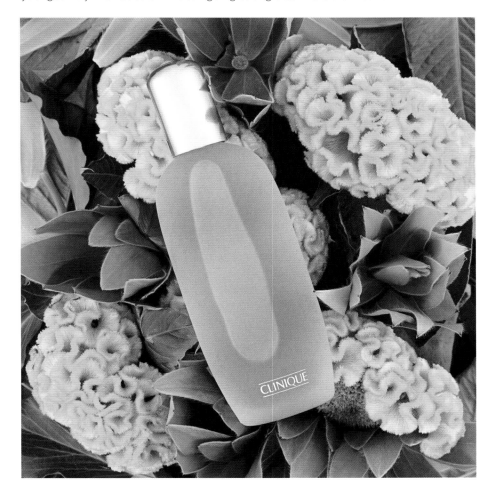

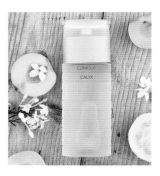

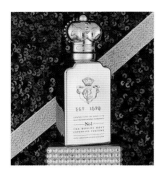

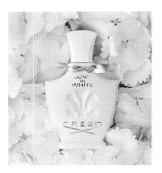

31 Clinique Calyx

Family: Floral
Launched: 1987
Creator: Sophia Grojsman

When Calyx burst onto the scene, a mega-trend was born – and floral-fruity fragrances still dominate the perfume universe today. In fact, this is one of the freshest, greenest, light-as-a-helium-balloon fragrances we've ever had the pleasure of encountering. Unmistakably, Calyx's first impression is a giant squirt of grapefruit – like plunging your nails into the peel of that fruit. Which turns out to be a fragrant illusion: there's no actual grapefruit in there. Instead, a cocktail of other fruits deliver that impression of juiciness: mandarin, passion fruit, apricot, peach, guava – plus bergamot and spearmint, for zing. Just when you start to think it's a fruit salad in a bottle, intense lily of the valley, freesia and slightly softer jasmine start to sneak prettily in. Allegedly, there's oakmoss, musk and cedar in the base – but for us, Calyx stays clear and enduringly fresh. Besides, most people we know who wear Calyx don't get to experience the dry-down much – because they're addicted to its zesty overture, and can't stop spritzing; its nose, Sophia Grojsman – one of the most commercially successful noses ever – also says she still sprays on Calyx when she needs cheering up and we completely understand why.

32 Clive Christian No. 1

Family: Floral
Launched: 1999
Creator: Unattributed

No. 1 makes the boldest of claims right on the crown-capped gold bottle: 'The world's most expensive perfume' (and is recognised by Guinness World Records as such). It was created without angst about the cost of the ingredients – and it certainly smells ultra-luxurious, particularly the whacking great bouquet of extravagant flowers at its heart: Indian jasmine, rose oil (6,000 a kilo), orris root (11,000), carnation, ylang ylang and more, with touches of fruit in there too: plum, pineapple and lemon. Seamlessly, the base notes then float in: an ambery vanilla roundness, with tonka, smooth sandalwood, cedar and musk. Clive Christian's own background is more than a little unusual: he designs and crafts the ultimate luxury kitchens and interiors for elite clients. Through the insights into the desires and lives of those clients, he knew that there was a market for truly opulent fragrances – and this is the first of several creations, all worth exploring, even if your budget's rather more IKEA, kitchen-wise. Even more luxurious bottles are available, including a half-litre Baccarat crystal flacon at $215,000. The website www.luckyscent.com is spot-on when it describes No. 1 as 'a first-class perfume ticket to a floral wonderland'.

33 Creed Love in White

Family: Floral
Launched: 2005
Creators: Olivier Creed and Erwin Creed

Gosh, this is unusual. You'd be forgiven for thinking the name Love in White was chosen to sum up a wedding-worthy bouquet of flowers – but there's much more going on here. The use of an unusual 'rice husk' note adds real intrigue to this creation from a family involved in perfumery for seven generations. It's inspired by Olivier Creed's 'ocean voyages' – and at a guess, in some of ports Olivier must have been presented with steaming bowls of white rice. Because that's just what you get in Love in White, alongside breaths of Spanish orange zest, daffodil (from the French Riviera), magnolia from the mountains of Guatemala, Italian jasmine and Bulgarian rose. Egyptian iris features, too, its creamy butteriness softening the whole composition beautifully. In the base, rejoin Olivier's voyage to be introduced to sensual notes of Mysore sandalwood, Javan vanilla and ambergris. Perhaps LiW's most significant geographical link, though, is The White House: the debut bottle was presented to Laura Bush and Michelle Obama is also said to wear it. You might not 'get' Love in White, at first sniff – but trust us: you'll keep coming back for another bowlful.

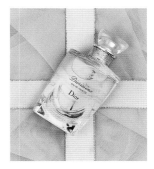

34 Dior Diorella
Family: Fresh **Launched:** 1972 **Creator:** Edmond Roudnitska

Diorella was the female counterpart to celebrated perfumer Edmond Roudnitska's masculine unisex fragrance Eau Sauvage (see page 151), sharing much of its glorious freshness: a first course of Sicilian lemon, peach, Italian bergamot and lemon, with a touch of basil, riding on a rocket-like 'zoosh' of aldehydes. It hardly sweetens at all – Diorella's essentially dry and airy – and the heart notes of jasmine and honeysuckle are elusive, like walking down a limestone-cobbled street and getting a whiff, just a whiff, of something pretty wafting in from a few gardens away. It becomes even 'greener', after a while: there's classic chypre oakmoss, but we can smell some labdanum, too – the so-green signature note also at the heart of Chanel No. 19. Base notes – which pleasingly hang around for ages on the skin – also include vetiver, musk, patchouli and sandalwood. You want to come across as a little bit enigmatic? Try wearing this: it's little-known, little-recognised (though truly, it ought to be) – and you'll definitely have them wondering what that glorious fresh scent you're wearing is. (You might have to stop the men in your life from snatching it away, though; this – like Eau Sauvage – is eminently borrowable.)

35 Dior Diorissimo
Family: Floral
Launched: 1955
Creator: Edmond Roudnitska

One of the greats. Truly, one of the greats – and like Indian tigers, at risk of extinction, if the 'authorities' have their way: the International Fragrance Association (IFRA) has been seeking a ban on the synthetic lily of the valley ingredient that bursts, soaringly, out of the Diorissimo bottle. We'll enjoy it while we can, then: pure, sweet, green gusts of lily of the valley, allegedly underpinned by ylang ylang and jasmine, sandalwood, rosewood and civet. (To be honest, we never get much except lily of the valley itself from Diorissimo, unless we close our eyes and really fish around for other notes – but who cares? Was there ever a more wonderful spring flower?) Diorissimo's creator, Edmond Roudnitska, was seeking to simplify his approach to perfumery, so we're told, and Diorissimo is the sensational result. It's crisp, sparkling, airy – but rich and intense at the same time, even in the eau de toilette form. (But oh, if you can get your hands on the parfum, let your senses wallow in that.) Diorissimo now resides within Dior's Les Créations de Monsieur Dior collection – and we recommend at least a brief encounter with each of them, actually, at Dior counters.

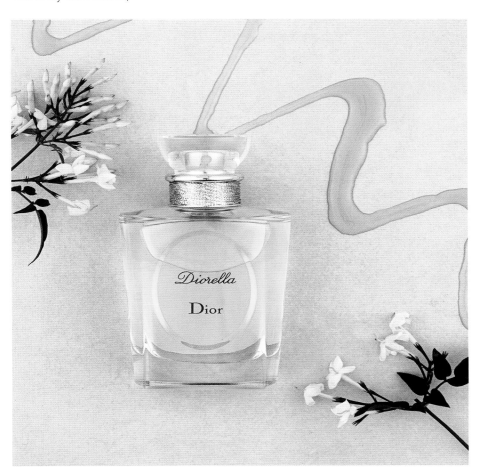

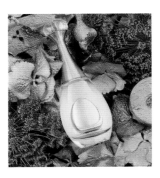

36 Dior J'Adore

Family: Floral
Launched: 1999
Creator: Calice Becker

Quite aside from having one of the most striking commercials ever made (if you haven't ever seen a gold-robed Charlize Theron walk through Versailles's Hall of Mirrors, get on to YouTube this minute), J'Adore is a total contemporary blockbuster. And fragrances only attain that status if something interesting's going on – which here means a peachy, pretty-pretty floral, as perfectly poised as the blondes who've advertised it over the years. At one count, there were apparently over 500 fragrances whose roots could be found in this radiantly fresh floral. It happens a lot in the perfume world: a 'bestseller' sets a trend and is then reinterpreted a gazillion times, usually with far less success. J'Adore is seriously fruity, at first – that peachiness, mandarin, and apricot, all juicy and summery. Then the floral notes swoop in, like a girl with her arms full of flowers: jasmine, rose, orchid (and a touch of plum). The fruit leitmotif continues through to the base, with a slightly tart note of blackberry, alongside soft musks and vanilla. It's amazingly long-lasting on the skin, glamorous but 'sunny' too – and packaged in what's become an iconic bottle, with its elongated, gold-ringed neck.

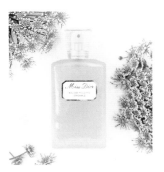

37 Dior Miss Dior *(Original)*

Family: Chypre
Launched: 1947
Creators: Paul Vacher and Jean Carles

On 12th February 1947, Christian Dior overnight made the wardrobe of every woman in the world look dowdy with the unveiling of his 'New Look': wide skirts fashioned from metre upon metre of fabric, with nipped-in waists, bare shoulders… Miss Dior was unveiled soon after – and women around the world swooned for it as they had Dior's full skirts. Miss Dior (the 'original' or 'classic', in contrast to the more recent Miss Dior Chérie) isn't exactly à la mode right now – but we long for it to be more widely known (and loved). It has a vintage quality, for sure: lots of galbanum-y greenness adding a dark twist to pretty-pretty rose, jasmine, neroli, narcissus, carnation and lily of the valley, which make for a soft, slightly powdery heart after you've been wearing Miss Dior on the skin. Humming beneath is a base of classic chypre notes, including oakmoss, patchouli and labdanum, a touch of handbaggy leather, some vetiver, sandalwood and ambergris for a velvety woodiness. Re-smelling it after too long an absence, we realise that this is as exquisite, polished and feminine a creation as ever – and really deserves to sweep the world once again.

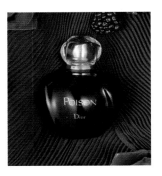

38 Dior Poison

Family: Floral
Launched: 1985
Creator: Edouard Flechier

Ker-pow! That was our reaction when we first smelled Poison at its launch in 1985 – at London's Hippodrome, with a ballet commissioned by the Dior parfums supremo Maurice Roger in celebration of its unveiling, and a going-home present (yikes) of a Poison-drenched hankie alongside the deep purple 'forbidden fruit' bottle. Even right slap bang in the middle of a decade of padded-shouldered, powerful scents, Poison was still an olfactory shock, with its massive dose of mentholly tuberose, berried top notes, OTT floral heart and s-e-x-y base: lots of vetiver, musk, vanilla and sandalwood (so tenacious they'll probably be on your skin until you next shower). Poison was the first fragrance launched by the house without the word Dior in its name and has since been followed by lots of what are known in the industry as 'flankers', including blockbuster Hypnotic Poison: enough of the original to attract devotees, but enough newness to seduce those who weren't previously fans. Poison is seriously intoxicating: you're not going to melt into the background wearing this, but even if you're not a lover of in-your-face fragrances, check it out as a landmark in fragrance history that endures to this day.

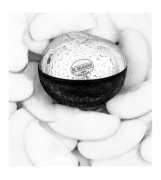

39 DKNY Be Delicious

Family: Floral
Launched: 2004
Creator: Maurice Roucel

Aside from anything else, you've just got to love the bottle: a perfect apple shape with a silver top, which you press to release a burst of this quintessential example of the floral-fruity family. (It's a pun on New York - the 'Big Apple', the NY of DKNY.) Many, many fruity-florals have come and gone – yet Be Delicious has become a 'keeper'. Probably because (despite the name, despite the bottle), it's more complex than just an apple scent. Actually, at first spritz, it's more cool-as-a-cucumber-y than apple scented. Then, for sure, a whole basket of apples whoosh in – not just the fruit (Golden Delicious, so the description goes), but sweet apple blossom. This fairly fleeting crisp green apple note is softened and balanced by delicate, petalled touches of lily of the valley, magnolia, violet, rose and tuberose – yet it stays sheer, clean and fresh, even as the base of white amber and woods develops later. We've given it to young perfume-lovers, who've gone into raptures over its very pretty yet crisp fruity floweriness – and who now buy every 'spin' on Be Delicious. (And there's been quite a harvest of those, thanks to the juicy global success of this original...)

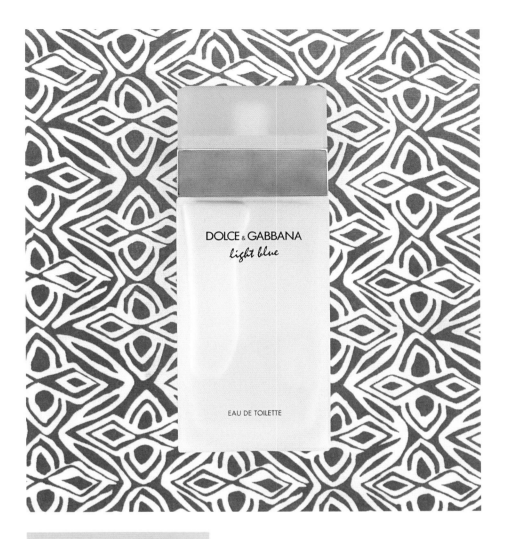

40 Dolce & Gabbana Light Blue

Family: Floral **Launched:** 2001 **Creator:** Oliver Cresp

Gosh, this is cheery and easy to wear – and you should, really you should. We're not surprised that at a time when there are as many as 1,100 fragrances launched each year, this creation by Olivier Cresp has stayed on the global bestseller list: it's like slipping on your favourite pair of jeans, which you know make you look and feel good. Only if this was a fabric, it wouldn't be denim: it would be something light and floaty, like organza, or maybe simply gossamer. There's a great open-window gust of airiness at the beginning, with the crunch of tart Granny Smith apple, Sicilian citron and a hint of bluebell (and aldehydes, we're guessing). A fragrance wouldn't be a fragrance without jasmine and rose at its heart, but they're here in the lightest dusting. And despite promising cedarwood, amber and musk among the base notes, it never goes too deep; of those, the amber comes through most clearly and it gets a little woodsy after a while. But Light Blue succeeds in staying sheer, radiant and refreshing right until the moment when you reach for the bottle and spray yourself all over again. As you will. You really will.

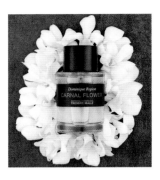

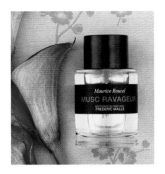

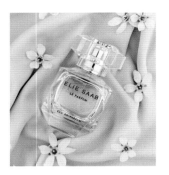

41 Editions de Parfums Frederic Malle Carnal Flower

Family: Floral
Launched: 2005
Creator: Dominique Ropion

You're either a tuberose-lover or you're not: it can be a touch headache-y, even with a hint of burning tyre. It may be divisive – but for tuberose fans, this Frederic Malle offering is the ultimate prize. Carnal Flower is reputed to have the highest concentration of any tuberose fragrance on the market – and everything else stays quietly in the chorus, allowing the flower the limelight. It's verdantly fresh at first, offering shimmering fruit touches of melon and bergamot. Eucalyptus adds almost a camphorous edge to the greenness, before the tuberose announces its presence in the perfume's heart and invites jasmine to dance. But the tuberose is leading the waltz here – and is light on its feet, which isn't always the way with what can be a seriously narcotic, heavy ingredient. The unexpected element is a touch of tropical coconut, which adds a gloriously milky sweetness, paving the way for soft, enveloping musk base notes. In India, young girls were warned against inhaling tuberose's aphrodisiac scent after sunset, in case it led them into trouble. Tuberose-lovers might choose to wear Carnal Flower, rather hoping for the same thing…

42 Editions de Parfums Frederic Malle Musc Ravageur

Family: Oriental
Launched: 2000
Creator: Maurice Roucel

Frederic Malle's decision to give some of the greatest perfumers on the planet free rein to create the perfume of their dreams, with none of the usual 'marketing brief' restrictions, unleashed a tsunami of creativity among those noses – including Maurice Roucel, who's behind this so-sensual composition. It's musky, for sure, right from the start – this is called Musc Ravageur, after all! – but all sorts of notes swirl seamlessly into one another in this subtle floral Oriental: animalic elements, amber, spicy cinnamon and cloves, sandalwood and vanilla, plus almost equally vanilla-esque tonka. And if that sounds cloying and headache-y, not a bit of it: lavender and bergamot brighten and lighten this work of art, but they're understated; there's none of the citrus 'whoosh' that bergamot generally delivers. (In fact, although top notes, heart notes and base notes are all mentioned, you really get the whole package from first glorious spritz.) 'Mellow' is the word that springs to mind when we smell this: soft, smooth, seductive – a sort of 'supper jazz' of a fragrance. Easy to slip into, comfortable to wear – and surprisingly 'shareable': we know lots of men who love and wear it.

43 Elie Saab Le Parfum

Family: Floral
Launched: 2011
Creator: Francis Kurkdjian

Orange blossom drizzled with honey. That's what you get when you unstopper this modern classic, which has done more to put Beirut-born fashion designer Elie Saab on the map than even his glamorous red-carpet gowns: his debut signature fragrance became an instant global bestseller on launch. (It's also won a slew of FiFis, the fragrance industry's own Oscars.) Many florals tend towards richness and heaviness: by contrast, this is sunbeams in a bottle, radiant, fresh and light-filled (thanks to lots of aldehydes). As the neroli floats away, other flowers drift in – the gardenia and jasmine that both flourish in Saab's home country, and a touch of rose: perfumer Francis Kurkdjian has beautifully captured the designer's own memories of the Mediterranean, in what's a very pretty faceted bottle. There's the eensy-weeniest trace of musk in the base, some patchouli and cedarwood – just enough to keep it tethered to planet Earth, but it is more chaste than carnal. The description given to Elie Saab Le Parfum perfectly sums it up: an 'ode to light'. That 'ode' is wearable to the office, we'd say – not intrusive, and 'clean' rather than cloying. But actually, it'd be just beautiful on a bride, too.

44 Escentric Molecules Molecule 01

Family: Woody **Launched:** 2006 **Creator:** Geza Schoen

A wild card, this. German perfumer Geza Schoen plays tricks not just on the perfume-lover but the whole industry with Molecule 01. Some people can't even smell it: they're 'anosmic' to the single note on which Molecule 01 is based, a synthetic called 'iso e super'. Others don't 'get' it straight away: iso e super is technically a 'base' note and may take time to unfold on the skin. Geza Schoen chose the note because it's also said to react with body chemistry, to create a pheromone-like effect. It certainly makes for as divisive a fragrance as we've ever encountered – which just makes it more interesting, we think. Some wearers (and yes, that does include us) experience a gently earthy, woodsy (especially sandalwoodsy) scent with fairy-breaths of vanilla, with a cool, metal edge at the same time – and it seems as if half the reviewers on sites such as Basenotes and Fragrantica can also smell it, and experience great longevity. The other half can't, and think it's little more than coloured water… Still others have tried it as a 'base' for other fragrances, to boost their sexiness (successfully, it seems). Emperor's New Clothes? Try it yourself and make up your own mind.

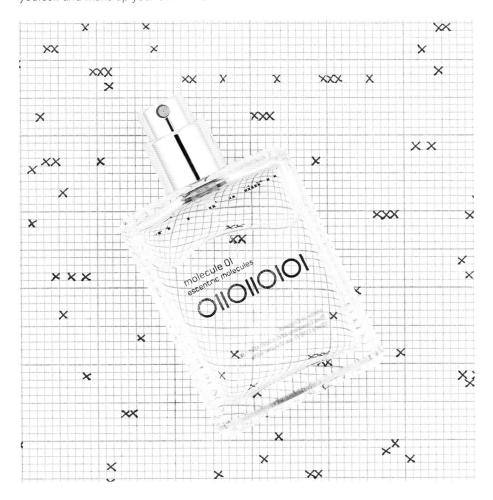

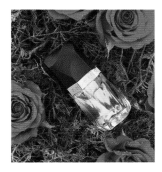

45 Estée Lauder Knowing

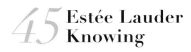

Family: Chypre
Launched: 1988
Creator: Jean Kerleo

Chypre fragrances are considered among the most 'sophisticated' creations. Nobody starts out wearing chypres: they're something you graduate to after the early, sweet-scented years – grown-up as a pair of patent high heels and a snap-clasp handbag. And Knowing is as elegant as fragrance gets: a rose chypre launched in 1989, just before the fad of less-is-more hit the perfume counters. It might seem like a throwback to the 1980s, but Knowing actually channels the old-school perfumery tradition of the 1920s and 30s: opulent, powerful, fusing plum, orange flower, jasmine, tuberose and mimosa around a rose heart – think: two dozen extravagant red roses, here – on a base with lots and lots of moss, a good slug of vetiver, just ever-so-slightly softened by sweet amber and rocket-propelled by patchouli. The French perfumer behind Knowing, Jean Kerleo, went on to become one of France's most acclaimed 'noses', working in-house at Jean Patou, before helping to set up France's Osmothèque perfume museum. A dab of this will do: apply last thing, after pinning on a big, bold brooch and before heading out the door – and we'd bet you'll have a little more sway in your sashay with Knowing.

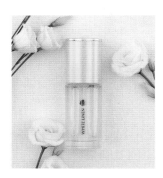

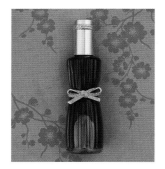

46 Estée Lauder White Linen

Family: Floral
Launched: 1978
Creator: Sophia Grojsman

What's in a name? Everything, for a perfume – and especially with this, which is as crisp and clean and fresh as it sounds. If your idea of heaven is smoothing away creases at an ironing board while your nose fills with fragrant steam, or you're crazy for the scent of sheets drying in the breeze, or if you just like to have the windows thrown open to allow the air to gush in at every opportunity, you'll love White Linen's outdoorsiness. The fragrance was created by one of the most famous 'noses' of all time (and a woman, at that), Sophia Grojsman. Aldehydes give the initial starchy 'rush', which is this fragrance's signature, along with citrus oils and a hint of peachiness. At the heart, though, are soft white florals: distinct breaths of lily of the valley, jasmine, iris, lilac and ylang ylang, alongside rose, all blurred seamlessly into one. This pure, absolutely perfect (and less-well-known-than-it-should-be) fragrance reflected America's love of all things 'clean' – and it's definitely romantic rather than sexy. The base notes merely whisper: cedar, amber, honey, tonka, benzoin and (allegedly) civet – but this is one for starched white shirt days, not smoke-filled speakeasies.

47 Estée Lauder Youth Dew

Family: Oriental
Launched: 1953
Creator: Josephine Catapano

Everyone should encounter Youth Dew – because this is the scent that changed the course of modern perfumery. Until this iconic Oriental came along, women didn't buy perfume for themselves but waited patiently for birthdays and Christmas. Estée Lauder's genius was to launch Youth Dew as a bath oil, which women didn't feel guilty about spending the housekeeping on. And a bath oil that doubled as a skin perfume would be acceptable to buy because it was feminine: all-American, very girl-next-door. We know many people who shy away from Youth Dew – for no real reason other than they know it's powerful stuff. Yes, it's exotic: a swirl of spices (cinnamon, clove), and opulent florals (ylang ylang, rose, jasmine). No, it's certainly not a shrinking violet: those base notes bustle in like a rowdy posse from the start, riding on an aldehydic wave (if aldehydes were good enough for Coco Chanel, Mrs Lauder reasoned…). They stay and stay and stay: resinous benzoin, patchouli, amber and tolu (a balsamic resin also used in cough medicine). But on the skin, allowed to unfold, we think Youth Dew is sublime – with an almost addictive soft amber-y warmth that lingers beautifully for aeons.

48 Etat Libre d'Orange Jasmine & Cigarette

Family: Woody
Launched: 2006
Creator: Antoine Maisondieu

Non-smokers, don't be put off by the name of this: it's a sophisticated floral in the style of Chanel No. 5 – but cleverly, the tobacco cuts through the sweetness of jasmine, adding depth and warmth. (We hate smoky rooms or even walking behind someone smoking on the street, but just love this; when used in fragrances, tobacco definitely has a honeyed, rather than an old-ashtray, quality.) The name might conjure up decadent nightclubs, but at its heart, Jasmine & Cigarette is sparkling and green, cheerful and summery, not heady and intense at all; the jasmine is there, but just a handful of sprigs rather than clambering rampantly over it. As a result, this scent is decidedly more lunch-party-on-the-terrace than after-dark party-wear. Niche perfume brand Etat Libre d'Orange break a lot of rules with their scents (and are fairly affordable for a 'cult' brand), but this – along with Fat Electrician (yes, that's really a fragrance name) – is our absolute favourite. It continues to smell sun-warmed in its 'dry-down': notes of tonka and musk sweeten and soften it, and you might – if your nose is tuned in – get a whiff of hay, like burying your nose in a haystack. Intriguing.

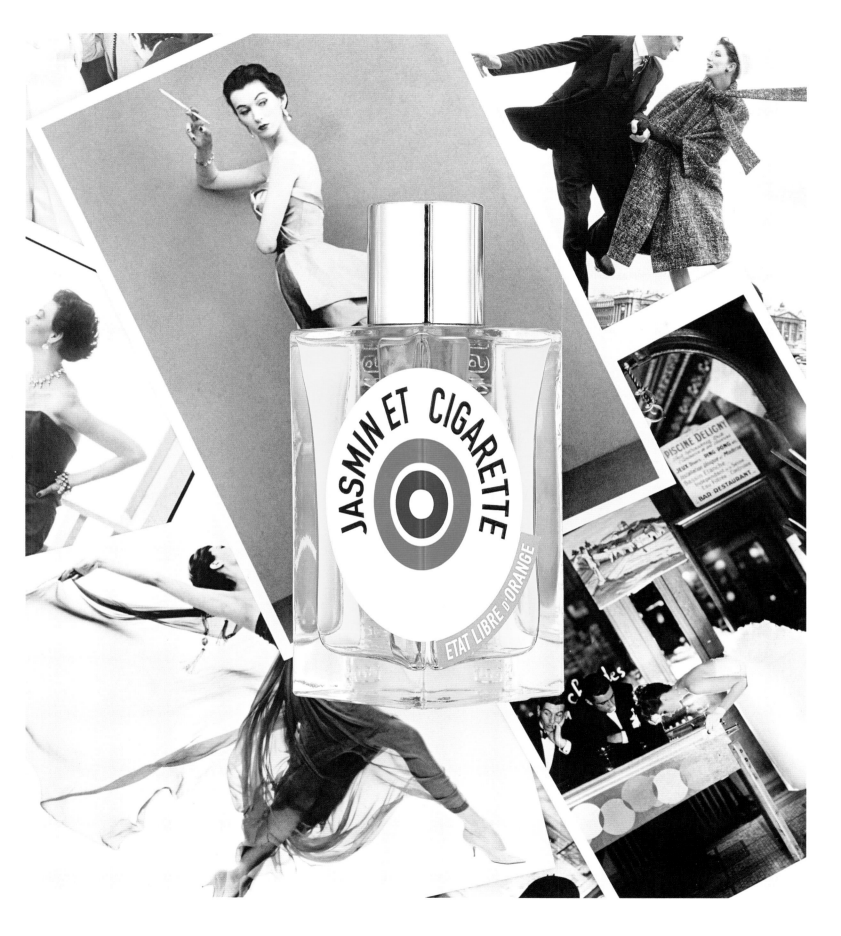

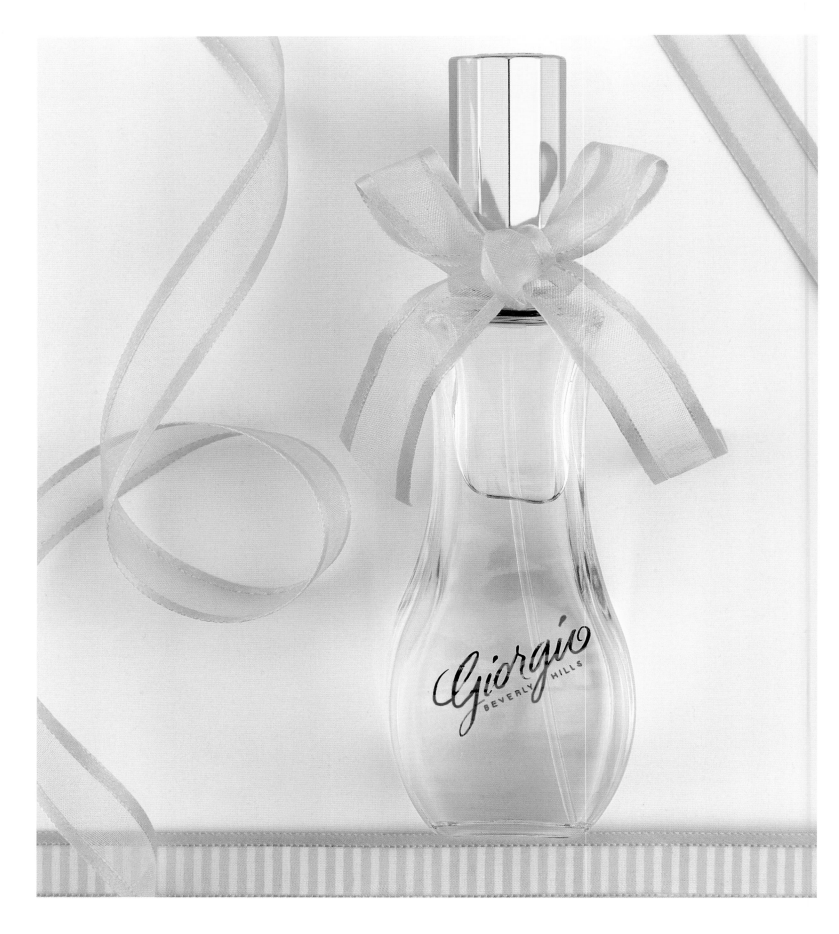

49 Giorgio Beverley Hills

Family: Floral
Launched: 1981
Creators: M.L. Quince, Francis Camail and Henry Cuttle

Giorgio was a landmark fragrance in all sorts of ways: it was the first ever to be advertised via a magazine 'scent strip', which introduced perfumistas to this fragrance through the glossy pages of magazines such as *Vogue*. It worked a treat: almost overnight, Giorgio took the perfume world by storm, becoming a massive bestseller. But Giorgio kicked up something of a stink, not long after: it was even banned in some restaurants and offices, for its sheer power. Yet when Giorgio is applied with the daintiest of touches, nostalgically we find it just so exquisitely pretty and feminine: wafts of orange flower and bergamot, at first, before the massive bouquet of white flowers swaggers in. Think: tuberose, rose, orchid, gardenia, jasmine – a bouquet the size an Oscar-winner might expect to have delivered by her film studio the morning after the awards. (And with a bowl of ripe peaches alongside.) This heart stays sunnily radiant for ages, the base notes almost understated by comparison: a sexy little combo of sandalwood, vanilla, amber, patchouli, oakmoss, cedar and musk, nonetheless. This really is glamour, bottled. But just a drop, remember. Just a drop.

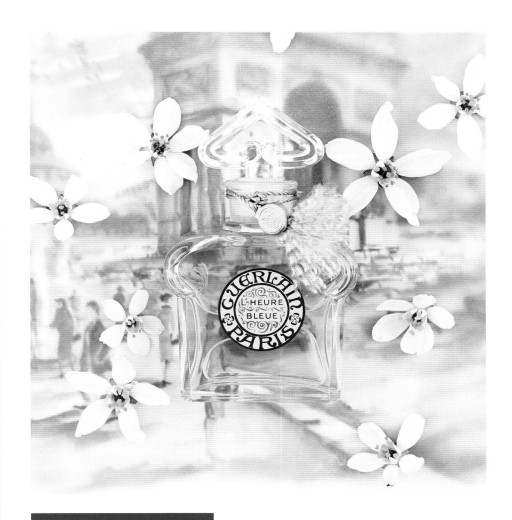

50 Guerlain L'Heure Bleue

Family: Oriental   **Launched:** 1912   **Creator:** Jacques Guerlain

L'Heure Bleue is a fragment of living fragrance history: it's survived two world wars and passed its centenary. So it's truly a fragrance that you can dab on to be transported back in time to a magical period in fragrance history, when third-generation family perfumer Jacques Guerlain was inspired to create L'Heure Bleue during a walk along Paris's La Seine, when he noticed the vivid, deep blue of the sky as dusk fell over Paris. 'I felt something so intense, I could only express it in a perfume,' he later wrote. It's an exquisite, plush scent, fusing the opulence of iris, ylang ylang and carnation and the sweetness of orange flower with sensually rich sandalwood, purring animalic notes (musk), incense, and delivering the exquisite powderiness of vanilla that is the signature of so very many Guerlain fragrances. Aldehydes – those dazzling, bright synthetics – give it ravishing radiance. L'Heure Bleue has great sillage: the quality that makes it waft around you so everyone else notices what you're wearing. (And probably swoons, over this.) Today, it's far less well-known than it should be – often tucked away at the back of Guerlain counters. Do, please, get a consultant to excavate it.

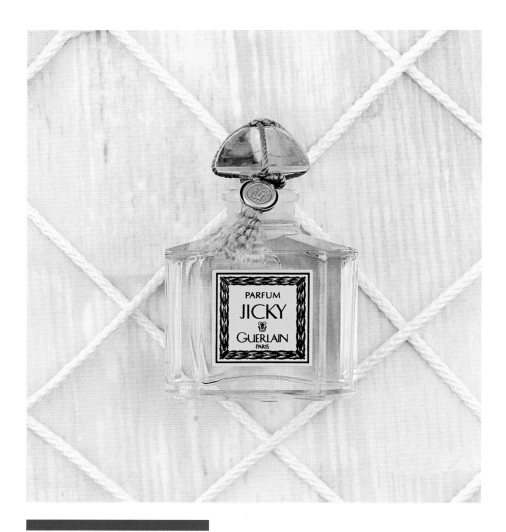

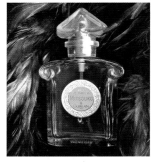

52 Guerlain Mitsouko

Family: Chypre
Launched: 1919
Creator: Jacques Guerlain

We love the idea that the great ballet impresario Diaghilev used to spray his curtains with this whenever he arrived in a new hotel. Because long, long before today's 'fruit-salad' fragrances – juicy with melon, raspberry and mango – were a twinkle in perfumers' eyes, there was Mitsouko. A soft, fuzzy peachiness drizzles honey over the opening breath of what is one of the greatest chypre fragrances ever created: Luca Turin says it's his favourite ever fragrance creation. And Jo's with him on that: it's the scent she returns to, winter after winter. What every creation in this fragrance family has in common is oakmoss, giving a damp, almost forest-floor intrigue to the classic rose and jasmine that (classically) twine round Mitsouko's heart, along with lilac. Labdanum (another chypre cornerstone), vetiver, patchouli and gentle, pulsing cinnamon and clove, meanwhile, deliver a really nuzzleable, snuggly quality to this masterpiece. If you used to adore Mitsouko but felt it had changed, then you're dead right: restrictions on oakmoss (a potential allergen) meant that its levels were reduced. Today, clever Thierry Wasser, Guerlain's current nose, has returned Mitsouko to its former glory.

51 Guerlain Jicky

Family: Oriental   **Launched:** 1889   **Creator:** Aimé Guerlain

Unveiled the year the Eiffel Tower was opened, Guerlain tells us that Jicky has been in production longer than any other fragrance. Initially, it was favoured by men. (And we know lots of men who still love and wear it today. Quite right too.) Pioneeringly, Jicky used the new synthetic perfume elements – coumarin and vanillin – along with a powerful dose of civet. Jicky broke with perfume tradition, too, through its complexity; previously, perfumes tended to be 'single note' or 'soliflores' (think: jasmine, rose, lavender). It packs a surprising lemon-y punch at first, before you encounter the vanilla-y coumarin, which fuses exquisitely with aromatic lavender. If you know the Guerlain portfolio, Jicky really couldn't be from any other brand, featuring generous quantities of their 'secret' Guerlinade, the blend of thyme and herbs and heaven knows what else, which gives almost every Guerlain creation an unmistakable signature. If you can possibly smell – or even acquire – the parfum, do. It will get you noticed – and ensure you are forever remembered. Luca Turin, author of *Perfumes: The A–Z Guide*, calls it 'a towering masterpiece', not a phrase he uses lightly – and we can't help but agree.

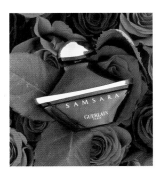

53 Guerlain Samsara

Family: Oriental
Launched: 1989
Creator: Jean-Paul Guerlain

Samsara was unveiled at the end of a decade of 'room-rocker' scents (see Giorgio, page 123), but this marriage of jasmine and sandalwood is more understated and quietly intriguing than many 1980s creations. Its back-story: for the very first time in their history, Guerlain decided to open up the creation of a new perfume to outside fragrance houses. Jean-Paul Guerlain entered the 'beauty parade' himself, though, with a creation he'd come up with to seduce an English girlfriend: a soft, creamy blend of Indian jasmine, rose, narcissus and ylang ylang, with bergamot greeting you brightly (and briefly) at the start. There's more sandalwood than most in Samsara, and if you love that pulsing base note, you may well fall head-over-heels for this: according to perfume expert Michael Edwards, it makes up as much as 30 per cent of the creation. On the skin, velvety hints of tonka and vanilla drift in to accompany the milky sandalwoodiness. (It's one of the only Guerlain fragrances not to include their signature 'Guerlinade' complex, though – which is why it's not as recognisable at 50 paces as some.) The bottom line? Jean-Paul Guerlain won the 'competition' for the new launch – and the heart of his lady.

54 Guerlain Shalimar

Family: Oriental **Launched:** 1925 **Creator:** Jacques Guerlain

Meet one of the world's most famous, most voluptuous, most recognisable fragrances. You've walked behind women trailing a Shalimar sillage – and every woman should do that herself at least once in her life. Jacques Guerlain believed vanilla was a great aphrodisiac, adding lashings to this fragrance (named after a famous garden in India, with a love story at its heart). Shalimar has a blink-and-you'll-miss-it bergamot moment before flowers bloom at its heart. But it's the so-sexy base – all warm benzoin, soft vanilla, come-and-get-me musks – that has women (and the men who like to get within nuzzling distance) coming back for more. We love this description from the Perfume Shrine blog: 'Shalimar's feminine beauty comes from the orchestration of its softly powder and animalic elements, that heave like an ample bosom…' Teenagers should not apply: every few years, Guerlain tries to 'reinvent' Shalimar for a younger audience – but we think this icon should remain something a woman grows into, along with an appreciation of the difference between prosecco and Cristal Champagne, say. Well, if Shalimar was a champagne, it would be Cristal – and we're equally happy to indulge. As often as possible, s'il vous plait.

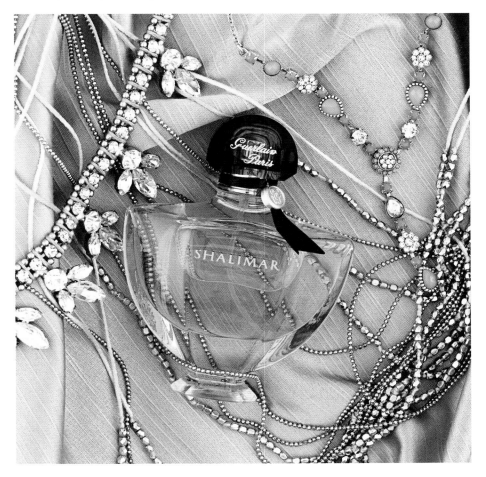

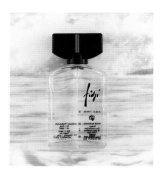

55 Guy Laroche Fidji

Family: Floral
Launched: 1966
Creator: Josephine Catapano

According to author and perfume expert Michael Edwards, Fidji 'pioneered a new generation of fresh perfumes', including Charlie (1973), Gucci No. 1 (1975), even Chanel No. 19 (1971) 'and a hundred other fragrances following its lead'. What made – makes – Fidji special? A fresh, slightly fuzzy beginning, with bucketfuls of green (even, occasionally, bitter) notes, including lemon and hyacinth, which contrast beautifully and pave the way for jasmine, Bulgarian rose, iris and ylang ylang. Allegedly the inspiration for Fidji was Nina Ricci's L'Air du Temps, but this was designed to have a way more youthful feel. However, if you're expecting tropical white flowers like tiaré or frangipani, or a South Sea Islands feel to Fidji, you're in for a surprise: this is heels rather than bare feet, a suit rather than a grass skirt, hair up rather than loose. On the skin, the green notes give way to the milky softness of sandalwood and musk, with vetiver and oakmoss helping to deliver an understated sexiness. Almost 50 years after its launch, Fidji still manages to be fresh and light, yet sensual and seductive, all at once – something of a multitasker, which would happily accompany you from desk to dinner.

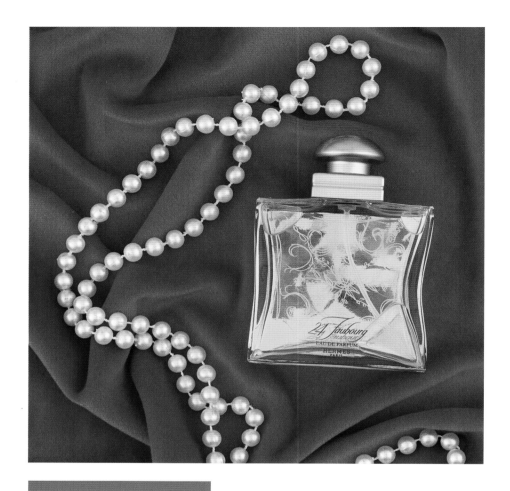

56 Hermès 24 Faubourg

Family: Chypre **Launched:** 1995 **Creator:** Maurice Roucel

Click, click, click. We can almost hear the high heels of the straight-backed, head-held-high woman in 24 Faubourg, doing the 'model walk' across the marble-floored foyer of a swanky Paris hotel: The Crillon, probably, maybe Le Meurice or even the Ritz itself. Actually, this is Paris, in a bottle – not the edgy Paris of artsy Bastille or bohemian Montmartre, but the city's money-no-object epicentre, where the world's swankiest boutiques sit shoulder-to-shoulder, luring luxury-lovers from all over the world. You want to smell – and consequently feel – elegant? Unstopper a bottle of übernose Maurice Roucel's masterpiece (should that be mistress-piece…?), and apply before your pearls, your diamonds (or your faux: when you wear this, nobody will think they're fake unless you spill the beans). Voluptuous doesn't even begin to cover it: jasmine, exotic tiaré flower, ylang ylang, with swags of pretty orange blossom – basically like one of those massive abundant floral displays you'd encounter in a 7-star luxury hotel. 24 Faubourg's chypre character emerges when it's been skin-warmed for a while. There's a sumptuous base of musk, amber, sandalwood, patchouli and deliciously damp mossiness, with plenty of sillage – the pulsing quality that ensures with this that you leave a divine scent-trail in your wake.

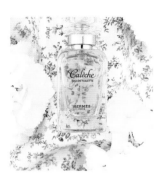

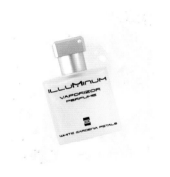

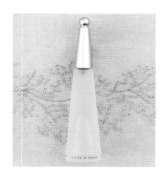

57 Hermès Calèche

Family: Floral
Launched: 1961
Creator: Guy Robert

A work of art. That's the only way to describe Calèche, which we've read described as 'a perfume for the woman who doesn't have to try too hard'. (And wouldn't we all like to be described that way…?) Calèche means horse-drawn carriage, in French – and Hermès opened in Paris in 1837 to sell bridles and harnesses. You could definitely wear this with a riding habit – or a summer dress. Or a pair of jeans, come to that: Calèche does have an effortlessness about it. Outdoorsily fresh at the start, this fast shapes up to become truly womanly, as the heart notes bloom. Think: roses, jasmine, ylang ylang and lily of the valley. But the potentially overpowering powdery femininity of that posy gets a clean edge from a touch of cypress: a ride-through-an-evergreen-woods note, which works as a counterpoint to keep Calèche nicely crisp. The base is on the dry side: frankincense, vetiver, sandalwood, just ever-so-slightly softened by amber and musk. Calèche rather hides its light under a bushel, with more famous floral-aldehydics such as No. 5 and Arpège grabbing the limelight. Smell it for yourself, give it a well-deserved moment in the sun – and admire Guy Robert's artistry.

58 Illuminum White Gardenia Petals

Family: Floral
Launched: 2011
Creator: Unattributed

The is the bestselling fragrance from an intriguing new brand, which boasts a Mayfair-based flagship 'Fragrance Lounge' as its unique HQ (see more on page 87). Why so? Because Kate Middleton – now The Duchess of Cambridge – apparently wore it for her wedding to Prince William, and since then royal watchers and lovers of pure white florals have been beating a path to Illuminum's door. Royal approval or not, it's a 'florabundant' find, with gardenia at its heart, woven into a fresh – and yes, bride-worthy – bouquet, alongside ylang ylang, jasmine and muguet. Before you reach that heart, though, White Gardenia Petals leads you through a green tunnel – an airy corridor, en route to the main event. Gardenia can be heady, sultry, even headache-y – but here, it's handled with a light and pretty touch. It's long-lasting and would definitely see you through the wedding and the reception. After a while, soft, musky base notes seep in, with touches of amber wood. Meanwhile, we can't recommend highly enough that you pay a visit to Illuminum (or one of their stockists) to be led by the hand through a 'Sensory Journey' to meet your perfect Illuminum scent-match. It's quite a trip.

59 Issey Miyake L'Eau d'Issey

Family: Fresh
Launched: 1992
Creator: Jacques Cavallier

For his very first launch, the Japanese designer had the idea to create something that basically smelled – and looked – like water: the pale, almost transparent freshwater 'juice' was quite revolutionary, and (literally) a breath of fresh air after the decade of the 'room-rocker' perfume. (Those are the perfumes – and we've all smelled them – that trumpet someone's arrival, fanfare their farewell and are still discernible in a lift long after the passenger has stepped out.) L'Eau d'Issey is super-light and airy at the beginning: lotus, freesia, a touch of rosewater, lushly soft and feminine – the type of scent that won't overwhelm anyone at an interview or a business meeting. And there's a definite place for those, in someone's fragrance wardrobe). At the heart is lily, peony and another white flower, osmanthus: so far, so pretty. But there's a dry base to L'Eau that lingers for quite a while on the skin, becoming subtly musky, with sandalwood and cedarwood alongside a 'clean' rather than a raunchy musk. The Zen-like bottle, by the way, was designed by graphic design genius Fabien Baron (who was also responsible for ck one a few years later) and has become a true icon in its own right.

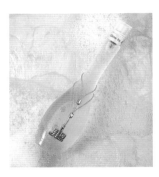

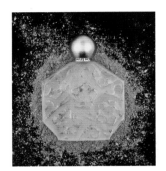

60 J.Lo Glow

Family: Floral
Launched: 2002
Creators: Louise Turner and Catherine Walsh

Celebrity scents have been the biggest fragrance 'trend' for more than a decade now – but this was one of the first, and may be around longer than most. Jennifer Lopez wanted of her debut scent 'something that feels like you just came out of the shower and you are the sexiest person in the world'. It obviously worked: this clean, somewhat soapy floral rang up over $100 million in sales in the first year alone, inspiring many other famous faces to dive headfirst into the scent market. Unlike some celebrity scents, though, it's pretty understated – and understatedly pretty, too. At first fresh – citrus and orange blossom are what you'll notice – it then morphs into a true floral, with a soft rosiness and an intriguing (not unpleasant) metal note. After a while on the skin, it becomes softly musky and nuzzleable and it has good staying power without being at all overwhelming. Glow has an intimacy: it won't intrude into the airspace around you unless someone gets seriously close. Trust us: it's quite lovely, a genuine, pretty foolproof classic that you could give to a daughter, a sister, a colleague – and be quite happy to wear yourself, come to that.

61 Jean Charles Brosseau Ombre Rose L'Original

Family: Floral
Launched: 1981
Creator: Françoise Caron

Lovely story behind this. Apparently, Jean Charles Brosseau – a French accessories designer – was visiting his fragrance manufacturer and fell head over heels for a fragrance sample which had been sitting on their shelf for years: it reminded him of his aunts, who were dusted to the nines on Sundays. And powdery this most definitely is: a nimbus, a froth, a haze of rosy-pinkness, perfectly echoed in the 'lingerie' tones of the juice itself. It's an unashamed posy of florals: lots of rose (the name means 'rose shadow'), ylang ylang, lily of the valley – but first, an overture of aldehyde-fuelled honeyed peachiness, with just a touch of aromatic geranium. It's true that it's a little old-fashioned, a touch soapy at times, but it's also angora-soft and feminine as fragrance gets. We're not sure you'd give it to an aunt: it would actually be a beautiful first fragrance for a young woman – something different to the usual 'celebrity' scents (most of which certainly won't be with us 30 years from now). One of the most delicious things about Ombre Rose is the bottle: originally designed for a 1920s fragrance called Le Narcisse Bleu, it's as 'vintage' as a modern perfume bottle gets.

62 Jean Patou Joy

Family: Floral
Launched: 1930
Creator: Henri Alméras

Launching a fragrance declaring itself to be 'the world's most expensive perfume' during The Great Depression certainly put Jean Patou on the map, with the couturier's Joy becoming the second bestselling fragrance of all time, behind No. 5, in its day. (Although we have a hunch that under the guidance of Thomas Fontaine, Jean Patou's new 'nose', Joy's return to glory is just around the corner). And oh, does it truly smell luxurious, embracing the wearer with the floral explosion of a harvest of 10,600 jasmine flowers and 28 dozens of roses at its heart, alongside tuberose, ylang ylang and iris. (Though the jasmine wins the war with the roses, we'd say.) It is proper grown-up womanly, beautiful, classic – perfectly balanced, with no harsh edges. As the flowers mellow, so the seductive base makes itself known: deep and complex and intriguing, lingering till morning on the skin. It's one for wearing to cocktails, or La Scala, or a wedding (very possibly your own, as white florals lend themselves beautifully to brides). Today, though, in a world of fabulously-priced niche fragrances, Joy is no longer even close to being the costliest on the market.

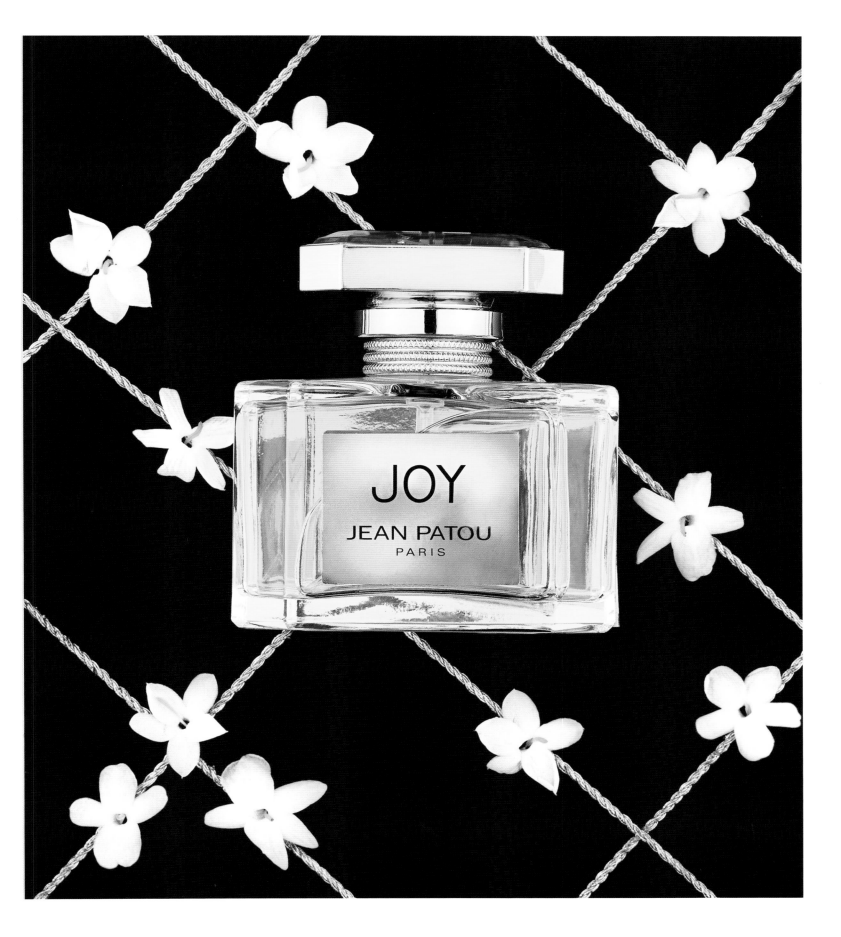

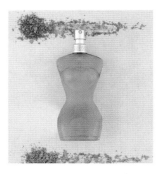

63 Jean Paul Gaultier Classique

Family: Floriental
Launched: 1993
Creator: Jacques Cavallier

Jean Paul Gaultier's brief to Jacques Cavallier was for a fragrance to conjure up his grandmother's dressing table, with plenty of powderiness and hints of the acetone you get in nail polish. At first glance that doesn't make for a promising start, but this sweet, powdery and long-lasting (in every way) debut scent from the irreverent French designer has truly become the 'Classique' of its name. It's as feminine as it's possible to imagine and, even now, it is not like anything else out there. First comes orange, cassis (a currant-y, berry-ish note), plum and peach. For that 'nail polish/pear drop' vibe, Cavallier used benzyl acetate, made more voluptuous by the inclusion of lots of ylang ylang, orange flower and fruity rose notes, and the warmth of ginger. The base? A big helping of vanillin, some iris and lots of powdery, woody-amber Ambrox, delivering a warm, soft, musky 'face powder' effect. The bottle's a stunner: it gives more than a nod to Schiaparelli's renowned tailor's dummy flacon for Shocking, but with a sexy corset etched onto the glass. The knicker-pink juice itself is the finishing touch to a fragrance that's sexy, sexy, sexy. And not a bit like most people's granny, frankly!

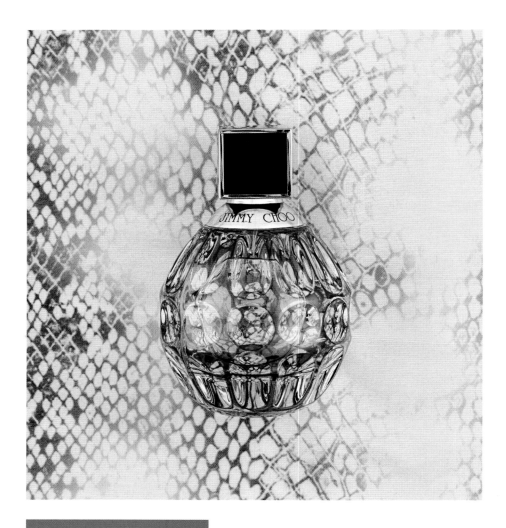

64 Jimmy Choo Jimmy Choo

Family: Chypre **Launched:** 2011 **Creator:** Olivier Polge

Jimmy Choo's shoes are (legendarily) amazingly easy-to-wear: footwear of choice for slinky-limbed aristos, WAGs and fashionistas. This scent is just as easy – and a lot more accessible for most of us than a pair of handmade, vertiginous stilettos. What you get at first spritz is a sherbety whoosh, which feels young, fresh, exciting – but then blink and it develops all the sophistication of a leather-lined limousine. Technically, Jimmy Choo's a chypre – considered the most elegant of fragrance types by many – but the vanilla's ramped up, and the fragrance has a delicious gourmand, almost salted caramel heart. Jasmine and tiger orchid feature – but the powdery, candied elements win out over the florals, in the heart-space. We like this best as it warms up on the skin: a fuzzy muskiness, little ambery whiffs, with vanilla tiptoeing in from the wings. Jimmy Choo is best enjoyed up-close-and-personal, purring quietly in the background. And as if the 'juice' itself wasn't desirable enough, the stunning grenade-shaped multifaceted Murano glass bottle (in the palest shade of lingerie pink) is beautiful. Any woman looks better dressed in Jimmy Choo, and any dressing table, better dressed, with a bottle of this new classic.

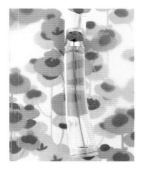

65 Jo Malone London™ Lime, Basil & Mandarin

Family: Fresh **Launched:** 1991 **Creator:** Jo Malone

Not too sweet, not too sour: just a mouthwatering, cooling balance of herby basil and sour lime, with touches of sweeter mandarin. Few Colognes make it to 'classic' status, but this acclaimed offering helped its creator – London-based facialist Jo Malone – build an entire fragrance empire, before selling it to Estée Lauder. (They've taken the fragrances to a whole new level of intrigue.) Effortlessly worn by men and women, it's clean, crisp, refreshing, uplifting, breezy: Lime, Basil & Mandarin doesn't quite effervesce in the bottle, but you can almost imagine it doing just that. Unusually, the Jo Malone London™ fragrance house is big on promoting the idea of 'combining' their perfumes, to create one-of-a-kind Colognes and perfumes just for you, but enjoyed on its own, this is like a long, cool drink of water on a hot day. Being mostly volatile citrus notes, it doesn't hang around on the skin for long – but that's a great excuse to keep re-spritzing and experiencing its zesty brightness time and again. (Jo Malone London™'s bestselling fragrance globally, Lime, Basil & Mandarin is available as home fragrance, too.)

66 Kenzo Flower by Kenzo

Family: Floral
Launched: 2000
Creator: Alberto Morillas

There are brazen in-your-face florals and soft-as-marshmallow florals and this, with its sort of baby-lotion fuzziness, falls into the second camp. There's a sensual powderiness to Flower by Kenzo: Mummy's face powder or a delicious body powder begging to be dusted onto just-bathed skin with a swansdown puff, maybe. Rose and violet, with their innocent softness, are generally considered a bit 'old-fashioned' by perfume snobs, who like their fragrances a bit edgy – but this actually smells modern rather than retro. Despite a generous dusting of vanilla, this is still lighter and airier than most Oriental florals but shares their addictive quality. (Rediscovering it, we found ourselves compulsively sniffing where we'd sprayed it. We also realised how often we'd smelt it when up-close-and-personal with female commuters on the Paris Métro.) White musk, opopanax, hedione (which evokes jasmine), hawthorn and cassia also feature. Since its launch, it has become one of the top-selling fragrances in Europe, hence plenty of variations on the Flower by Kenzo theme, launched by the brand to tap into its popularity (a summer version, a spiced-up spin) – but this remains our favourite.

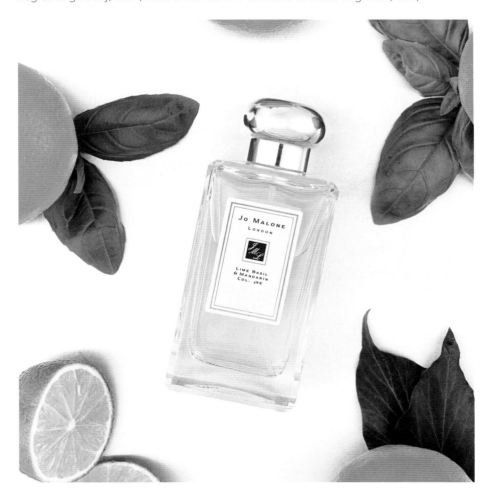

the perfume bible

131

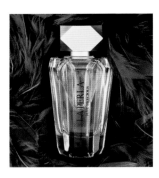

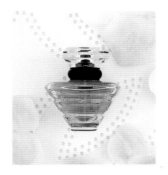

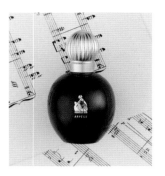

67 La Perla
La Perla

Family: Chypre
Launched: 1987
Creator: Pierre Wargnye

Chypre-lovers – if you aren't intimate with this smooth, rich, polished-to-perfection creation, you could just be on the verge of A Big Love Affair. (We think it belongs right up there with the chypre classics such as Mitsouko, Paloma Picasso and Sisley Eau du Soir.) When any lingerie brand launches a fragrance, of course (as Agent Provocateur and Victoria's Secret did decades later), the anticipation is that it'll be seductive and sensual – and La Perla truly delivers. (Definitely in a black lace rather than a white lace fashion.) The so-classic chypre notes of bergamot, rose, labdanum, patchouli and oakmoss are exquisitely balanced and then drizzled with a sort of honeyed softness. As time wears on, the woodiness in La Perla's base becomes more obvious: sandalwood, vetiver, patchouli, with touches of incense. Though it stays around on the skin for hours, La Perla doesn't muscle itself into a room's airspace as bossily as some classic chypres and we're hard-pushed to think of a better introduction to get acquainted with this refined family of fragrances. Perfect for a seductive rendezvous. (And to do it credit, you really should reach for your best underwear, rather than your good old Bridget Joneses.)

68 Lancôme
Trésor

Family: Floral
Launched: 1990
Creator: Sophia Grojsman

The 1990s was an 'understated' era, perfumery-wise – but although this crowd-pleaser was created at the start of that decade, Trésor definitely harks back to the 'room-rockers' of the 80s. It's packed with the fuzzy nectar of apricots and peach, romantic armfuls of white, fruity roses, iris and vanilla-y heliotrope: as a perfumer, Sophia Grojsman helped to pioneer mouthwatering combinations of fruit and flowers, setting a trend that is going as strong as ever, today. It's so iconic that *The New York Times*'s former 'Scent Critic' Chandler Burr chose Trésor as a key element of his 'Art of Scent' exhibition at New York's Museum of Arts and Design: visitors got the opportunity to smell the scent at different stages of its development, before this final version was launched to widespread acclaim. At the heart of Trésor is an accord Sophia code-named 'cleavage', which smells (so she says) like a young woman's décolletage. Smouldering beneath are notes of sandalwood, musk and vanilla, making for long-lasting application and a quietly pulsing sexiness. If you enjoy the scent of lipstick, or that 'Mummy's handbag' smell of face powder, if you like your fragrances as feminine as can be, this is a can't-fail choice.

69 Lanvin
Arpège

Family: Floral
Launched: 1927
Creator: Andre Fraysse

There are parallels between music and fragrance: for a start, they are both composed of notes and harmonies. Arpège is probably the most musically linked of all: the idea behind its composition is individual notes played one after another, rather than simultaneously. Arpège was a pioneering 'designer' fragrance, from couturier Jeanne Lanvin (famous for gorgeous, drape-y gowns). Lanvin dedicated this to her musician daughter – naming it Arpège, after the musical term arpeggio. If it was a piece of music, it would probably be a Mozart concerto. But just how does Arpège smell? Ravishing: sexy as a black velvet dress, very soigné. The almost champagne-like fizz at the beginning segues softly from citrussy bergamot to soft orange blossom, from rose to iris, jasmine to ylang ylang and so on: a delicious play on white flowers, which quietens down as the base notes of sandalwood, vetiver, vanilla, musk and patchouli continue to hum on the skin for hours. This isn't – precisely – the Arpège your great-granny might have worn for a night at the opera: in 1993, it was 're-orchestrated' by Hubert Fraysse (a descendant of the creator) – but with the greatest respect to its classical roots…

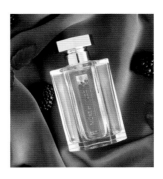

70 L'Artisan Parfumeur Mûre et Musc

Family: Floral
Launched: 1978
Creator: Jean-François Laporte

A fruit bowl of notes has made its way into perfumery in the past decade or two, but at the time it was pretty daring for Jean-François Laporte, the man behind L'Artisan Parfumeur, to weave tartly juicy blackberry through this early 'star' in L'Artisan's perfumed portfolio. And who'd have guessed it would pair so incredibly well with sultry, sexy musk, the inky sweetness drizzling jammily over that animalic note…? (The scent equivalent of combining basil with tomato in cooking, as Bois de Jasmin's blog cleverly observes – and a stroke of genius.) It all starts with the breeziest of beginnings, though: a wake-up call of aldehydes, ushering in Mûre et Musc's berry harvest, with a touch of orange blossom nodding alongside. Unlike the fruit-salad-y fragrances, which have topped the charts more recently, though, this stays crisp and green, rather than toppling over into sweetness. We love that it stays tart and fresh on the skin for hours, even as the vanilla drifts in: as indelible as a blackberry stain on your white T-shirt. (If you're on the prowl for your first whiff of Mûre et Musc, meanwhile, do also check out the exquisite 'Extrème' version, created by Karine Dubreuil…)

71 Liz Earle Botanical Essence No. 15

Family: Oriental **Launched:** 2012 **Creator:** Alienor Massenet

Traditionally, Oriental scents have been over-the-top sexy, heady and best suited to being accessorised by velvet, satin (or simply naked flesh…). This is 'Oriental lite' – more snugglesome than come-ravish-me, and with a delicious fuzziness round the edges. (Think: angora sweater or cashmere wrap.) It's the second scent from much-loved skincare brand Liz Earle: her Botanical Essence No. 1 is among our favourite fresh fragrances – and we've hardly met a woman who doesn't love it – but this is more complicated: a blend of 15 botanical ingredients (hence the name), and mostly, though not 100 per cent, natural. Pink pepper and bergamot are the 'fresh' opening elements in this 'fresh Oriental', and if you sniff carefully you might pick out a touch of rose at the heart. But mostly, No. 15 is a swirl of spices and woods: guaiac wood (sort of smoky and dry at once), clove, sandalwood, cedar and patchouli. Tonka bean, benzoin and Bourbon vanilla all add sweetness, yet without being sickly. It's probably a bit 'bottom-heavy' in terms of notes – but that just makes for impressive staying power; we can still smell it on our skin, next day. And like it all the more, for that.

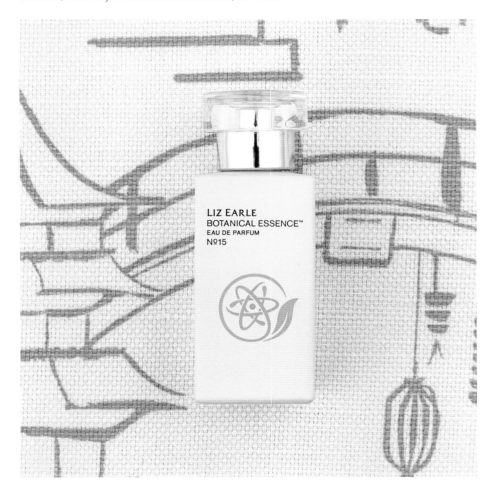

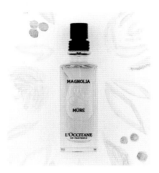

72 L'Occitane en Provence La Collection de Grasse Magnolia & Mûre

Family: Oriental
Launched: 2013
Creators: Karine Dubreuil and Olivier Baussan

First, we all knew L'Occitane as a bath-and-body brand. Then, following the global success of their Immortelle anti-ageing line, they became a skincare brand, too. But for us this is L'Occitane's most exciting incarnation of all, as they move into the world of fine fragrance – even going so far as to appoint Karine Dubreuil, Grasse-born 'nose', as their in-house 'composer', to underline their seriousness about this new adventure. La Collection de Grasse kicked off with a quartet of loveliness (three feminine fragrances, one shareable), of which this tart, blackberry-ish creation is our favourite. There's a twist of lime over the berries, to kick off, which contrasts well with the sweetness of magnolia, and lots of rose. (If you are lucky enough to bury your nose in a magnolia in springtime, some varieties have a berry-ish quality – so the pairing's pretty perfect.) Despite a woodier 'dry-down', with plenty of patchouli, Magnolia & Mûre stays pleasant and light throughout: one for sunny days, or for successfully conjuring them up when it's gloomy out there.

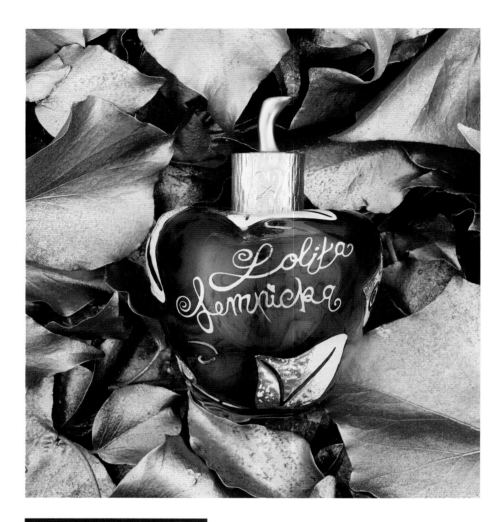

73 Lolita Lempicka Lolita Lempicka

Family: Gourmand **Launched:** 1997 **Creator:** Annick Menardo

Liquorice? In a fragrance? Absolutely: that saltiness is partly what makes Lolita Lempicka such a stand-out, among gourmand fragrances. Fragrance critic and molecular biologist (!) Luca Turin describes Lolita as a 'herbal Angel', and it certainly follows in Angel's footsteps, sashaying boldly into the pâtisserie: candied cherries, caramels, cotton candy. Yet it's somehow rather refreshing, too: not all sickly-sweet-sugary-prettiness, at all. We think of it rather like a salted caramel of a scent: the salt intensifies the sweetness, and vice versa. Like Angel, there's a decadent dose of dark patchouli and, well, shed-loads of vanilla in the sensual base of Lolita Lempicka (as well as some tonka bean, musk and vetiver). But before you step through the dark velvet curtains to arrive at that point, the note of liquorice (and anise, which isn't a million miles from liquorice) work along-side ivy leaves, as a balance to the edible notes of Amarena cherry and praline. A green floral note of violet helps lift things, too. The bottle is adorable, by the way – though why a mauve, gold-topped apple was chosen for Lolita Lempicka, we're not sure; despite featuring lots of gourmand ingredients, there's not a hint of apple in there…

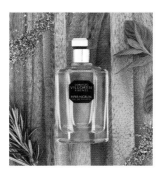

74 Lorenzo Villoresi Piper Negrum

Family: Oriental
Launched: 1999
Creator: Lorenzo Villoresi

There are many reasons to make a perfume pilgrimage to the city of Florence but Lorenzo Villoresi's fragrances are definitely right up there with the best of them. In Piper Nigrum, this independent Italian perfumer – who you can read more about on page 97 – weaves a tapestry of herbs and spices: not only black pepper (hence its name), but oregano, marjoram, nutmeg, rosemary, wild anise, dill and fennel – a bit like opening your herb cupboard and breathing in the coolness of mint and green herbs. But here's the thing: as one reviewer put it, Piper Nigrum is strangely 'warm and chilly at the same time' – and it's all the more interesting for that, we'd say. Because when it's given time to develop on the skin, Piper Nigrum actually becomes something of a hot water bottle of a fragrance; warm, spicy, enveloping (and as a result, ultimately more suited to cold nights than hot summer days). It even more interesting – and very, very seductive – as it develops on the skin into a creamy base of amber, styrax, benzoin, myrrh, Atlas cedarwood and a further sprinkling of spices. Gorgeous on women, sexy on men; we predict you'll be fighting over this bewitchingly unusual creation.

75 Maison Francis Kurkdjian Oud

Family: Woody   **Launched:** 2012   **Creator:** Francis Kurkdjian

Oud can be a love-it-or-hate-it ingredient – but even if you're not usually attracted to this traditional Arabian perfume ingredient (derived from a very special type of rotted wood!) – give this a go. Francis Kurkdjian is an astonishingly gifted perfumer and creator of global blockbusters including Jean Paul Gaultier Le Male and Narciso Rodriguez for Her – who also has his own glorious perfume house (read more about that on page 89). To be honest, we can hardly tell there's oud in here, so it's one for oud-refuseniks: it's soft and sweet, complex and wearable without being at all overpowering, almost more of a gourmand fragrance, with its edible qualities, than truly woody. Francis spices this up with a touch of saffron, and although the ingredients list doesn't acknowledge any flowers, there's a soft rose caress at the heart of this, which lasts for hours. We get sandalwood and cedarwood in the base rather than the famously animalic, often sweaty-smelling Arabian wood. (Soft touches of patchouli, too.) Oud's been one of the biggest trends in perfumery in recent years – a nod to the Middle Eastern consumer (it's not unusual for them to own 170 fragrances) – but this is one of its prettiest incarnations.

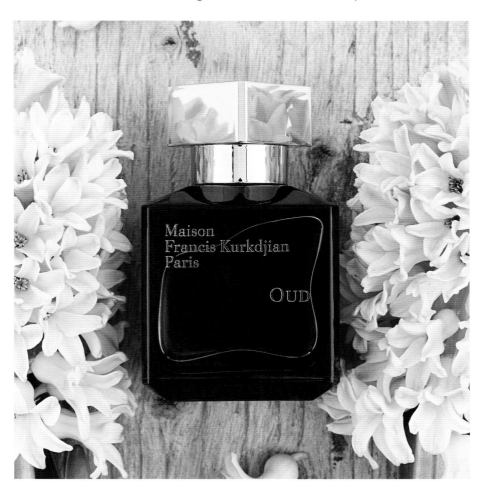

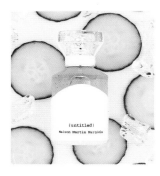

76 Maison Martin Margiela (*Untitled*)

Family: Woody
Launched: 2010
Creator: Daniela Roche-Andrier

Cool as a cucumber. Cool as crisp linen sheets. Cool as an ice cube, drizzled over sun-sizzled skin. We're always amazed at how some perfumes seem to have a 'temperature' all of their own – and this perfect summer spritz is definitely on the chilled side. But this also has a 'colour', too – and it's green, green, green. Close your eyes and sniff, breathe in the mossy mid-notes and the buchu – a relative of blackcurrant. We're right there in a shaded wood, lying on slightly damp ground, looking up into a leafy canopy. This creation from a Belgian designer known for his 'edgy' clothes took the fragrance world by surprise, becoming a major success. It has a squirt of grapefruit and mandarin in the opening and lots of orange blossom. Then curly mint – but in a dry, aromatic rather than a toothpaste-y way; it's at this moment that the green notes ricochet in, beckoning you deep into its chlorophyll heart. Then it goes all dreamy and airy and soft, and stays that way. Like Martin Margiela's designs, this belongs on someone who's comfortable in her skin. (Or his; we'd happily smell this on a man…)

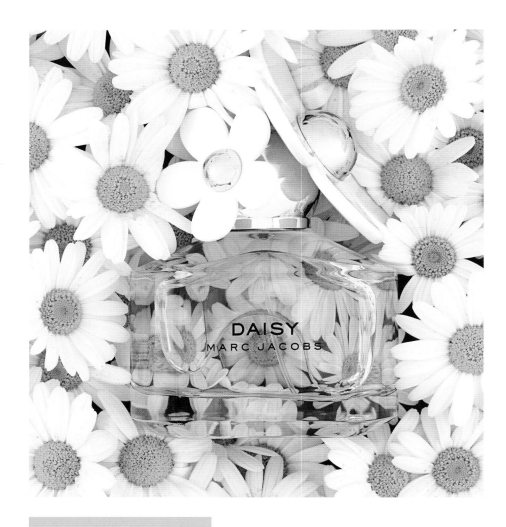

77 Marc Jacobs Daisy

Family: Floral **Launched:** 2007 **Creator:** Alberto Morillas

This fragrance put designer Marc Jacobs seriously on the global scent-map. 'Designer' fragrances, of course, have always been aspirational: can't afford the bag or the jacket…? Well, you can spring for the scent. But Marc Jacobs's scents are a phenomenon: total blockbusters, which also please the 'scent critics' of this world for their sheer, wearable prettiness. This scent has a squeeze of fruit at first sniff: grapefruit and wild strawberry, but with a transparent, aquatic quality – sheer as organza or chiffon. Violet leaves add a cucumber-greenness, as the scent segues into its floral heart: jasmine, gardenia, violet – sweet, but understated. Sunny and very upbeat, the white flowers are used with the lightest of touches and the base is equally whispering. If you wanted to cheer yourself up on a gloomy day, this should do the trick brilliantly. Youthful and vibrant, it would make a perfect present for anyone tentatively discovering the joys of fragrance wearing, although we know plenty of women of 'un certain âge' who love Daisy. Since this product, Marc Jacobs's bottle designs have become increasingly over-the-top, but with its vinyl daisy cap, this looks just as lovely on the dressing table as it smells on the skin.

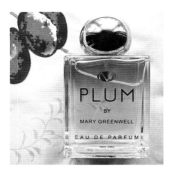

78 Marni Marni

Family: Woody **Launched:** 2012 **Creator:** Daniela Roche-Andrier

Fashionistas were on tenterhooks awaiting the debut fragrance from Marni – the colourfully chic-but-quirky Italian fashion brand, which has always marched to the beat of its own drum. We don't think anyone expected such a universally well-received yet soft-spoken fragrance, which had bloggers and beauty editors in raptures, frankly. Start with the stunning bottle: Marni-esque dots etched into hefty glass, with a cheerful splash of red on the cap. Then Marni turned to mega-talented perfumer Daniela Roche-Andrier for the 'juice' itself – also responsible for Martin Margiela (Untitled) and Prada Candy – and here's another cracker. It's pure sweetness and light, evoked by notes of bergamot and two kinds of pepper (pink and black), a twist of ginger, together with spicy touches of cinnamon bark and cardamom. Marni has a rosy-posy heart, but it's the base notes that truly beguile, wafting the softest trails of incense at you, delivering a lingering spiced powderiness on the skin. Marni's a year-round scent: light enough for warm summer days, just snuggly enough for cold weather. It's not overtly girly, despite the rose, fitting designer Carolina Castiglioni's brief for 'more of a masculine fragrance, with a touch of femininity'. As we like to say: discover, explore, enjoy.

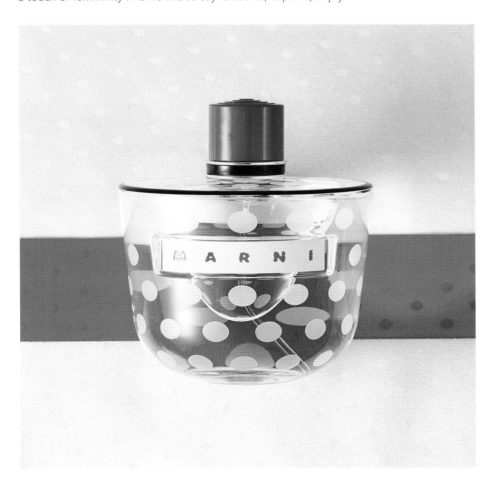

79 Mary Greenwell Plum

Family: Chypre
Launched: 2013
Creator: François Robert

This scent was quite some debut from a make-up artist better known for whisking her brushes across the faces of Cindy, Christy, Naomi, Claudia and Linda. At the time, we described it as 'Rich as Onassis, intense as Einstein, bold as Lady Gaga' and nothing much has changed, except that Plum has been widely acknowledged as a masterpiece. Its creator is François Robert, a fourth-generation perfumer with a fabulous pedigree (his father created Madame Rochas and Dioressence, while his grandfather Henri was responsible for No. 19 and Cristalle during his tenure at Chanel). Lush top notes are fruity without being too sweet: the plum of its name, a Bellini-ish dash of peach, classic citrus notes and blackcurrant. And then the heart literally folds round you like a slanket: gardenia, rose, jasmine and orange flower absolutes, with an understatedly exotic touch of tuberose. The heart notes linger and linger, but eventually base notes sashay sexily in: the classic oakmoss signature of a chypre, with patchouli, amber and white musk. Seriously, seriously sophisticated, the whole fah-bu-lous fusion – and with staying power worthy of the Duracell bunny. A star is born.

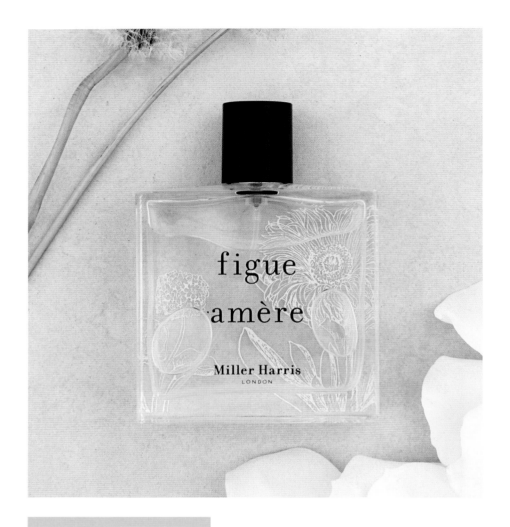

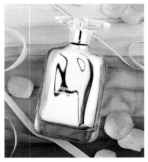

80 Miller Harris Figue Amère
Family: Floral **Launched:** 2002 **Creator:** Lyn Harris

A few years back, there was a major figgy trend going on: 'figmania', one blogger called it. But this – from British 'nose' Lyn Harris – has transcended fragrance fashion to become a true (unisex) classic, with a pleasingly green, almost bitter edge that's the perfect antidote when you're 'sweetied' out by gourmands, say. The fig's actually pretty understated in this, which is enticingly citrus-fresh at the start (mandarin and bergamot). Any bitterness of figleaf is softened by narcissus and rose – but then intriguingly accented again by another 'green' weapon in the perfumer's armoury: violet leaves, as well as galbanum from another Mediterranean plant, cistus, or 'rock rose'. Which, like figs, flourishes in very inhospitable, dry landscapes.) In the base, there's a sweet touch of amber, cedar and hints of moss. Yet there's somehow a salty breeze that wafts through Figue Amère too and after a while, it settles languidly down to become soft and sunny… If a perfume could capture 'lazy afternoons' in a bottle, this is it. Best enjoyed with a glass of chilled rosé on a terrace, overlooking blue seas, we say – or spritzed whenever that's exactly what you'd like to conjure up, on a more humdrum day.

81 Narciso Rodriguez Essence
Family: Floral
Launched: 2009
Creator: Alberto Morillas

This tactile 'mercury glass' bottle is one of our very favourites from recent years: the second scent from designer Narciso Rodriguez, and equally as feminine as his first. One of our favourite descriptions is from the Now Smell This blog: 'a hot steam iron pressing a linen dress that had been stored with a sachet of dried flower petals'. But she was damning this fragrance with faint praise, whereas we think it's super-pretty and super-appropriate for outdoorsy weekend days, or for subtle at-desk spritzing, or even for wearing to an interview if you wanted a little fragrant confidence boost but didn't want to knock out your future employer with anything but your intelligence. There's nothing blatant about Essence: aldehyde-fuelled petals, from velvety iris, rose (and a posy of white flowers). Yes, it has a fleeting 'scented drawer liner' moment, but Essence really gets interesting when it 'dries down', allowing the soft, sensual musk and amber to drift in. Then it develops a soothing, 'skin-scent' intimacy – really only to be enjoyed by someone who gets within nuzzling distance. If you like your musks clean and on the powdery side, rather than down-and-dirty, it's a must-try.

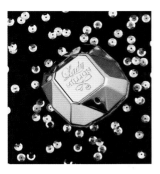

82 Nina Ricci L'Air du Temps

Family: Floral **Launched:** 1948 **Creator:** Francis Fabron

A gorgeous, blowsy bunch of flowers, this – and with a suitably romantic story. The bird on top of the L'Air du Temps bottle is a dove, symbolising peace: this so-feminine scent was created in the aftermath of the Second World War. Nina Ricci was one of newly-liberated Paris's legendary couturiers and her son Robert was the driving force behind L'Air du Temps's launch, working with perfumer Francis Fabron. Based on just 30 ingredients, it starts with a fresh whoosh, softening swiftly to its signature powdery sensuality – lots of iris, gardenia and jasmine. Hints of lush peach, sandalwood, amber, and the merest whisper of vetiver emerge over time. Look for super-collectible vintage Lalique bottles at flea markets: designed by Christian Bérard, this was declared 'Bottle of the Century' in 1999. Flacons still turn up and, if you unstopper the dove, you may get a breath of its former floral magnificence; many people say that L'Air du Temps has lost some of its grandeur over the years and it's certainly subtler than we remember – maybe more of a posy than a bunch, actually – but still beautiful. And wearable, too, on a first date or even a day at work.

83 Paco Rabanne Lady Million

Family: Floral
Launched: 2010
Creators: Anne Flipo, Dominique Ropion and Béatrice Piquet

'Sexy and sophisticated', chorus most of the online raves for this global blockbuster from Paco Rabanne, from the above trio of prominent 'noses'. It's a fruity floral, almost a scent cliché now that a gazillion have been launched in the past decade (they keep on coming), but it's got more going for it than most. Not least among its virtues is the striking gold 'diamond' spray bottle. With fragrance, you're meant to 'judge a book by its cover' – the bottle's a key part of the whole glamorous package – and this shrieks 'rich', which is an apt description for the scent inside, too. Raspberry and bitter orange are served up alongside neroli, in the top notes, and in the heart there's a more intense concentration of orange flower absolute and a great, intense bunch of jasmine, gardenia, peony and rose: elegant, luscious (and powerful). Among Lady Million's qualities is that it really clings to skin; that rich floral accord is the equivalent of a marathon runner, only gradually fading into a base that expertly balances notes of patchouli and musky woods with honey and vanilla. Best accessorised with very high heels, a beautiful frock and your best jewellery.

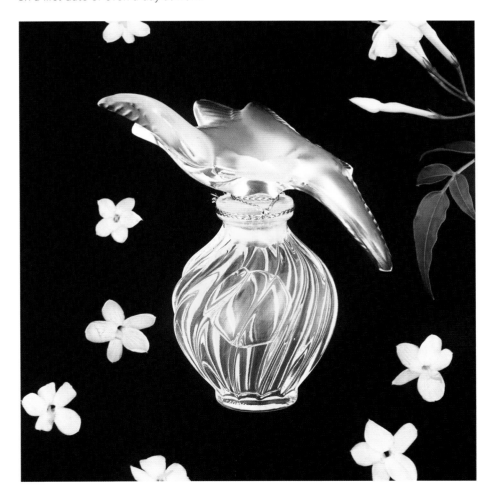

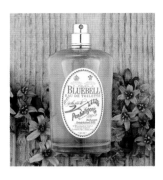

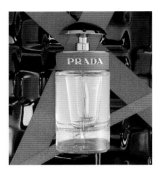

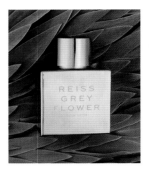

84 Penhaligon's Bluebell

Family: Floral
Launched: 1985
Creator: Michael Pickthall

Isn't one of the prettiest sights in the world a bluebell wood, in full bloom? Well, this is indeed rather as if the perfumer crammed an entire spring wood into the bottle. Bluebell is from British perfume house Penhaligon's, which dates back to the 1860s; William Henry Penhaligon later became Court Barber and Perfumer to Queen Victoria. Lately, Penhaligon's has become much more contemporary, with some stunning creations – but with nearly 30 years under its elegant belt, Bluebell is now in the realms of their classics. It's very green, at first – wow, it's green! – but then the heart notes of lily of the valley, hyacinth and jasmine make their presence felt. There's dewy rose, too – and a hint of spice from clove. We like its final phase: yet more greenness, from galbanum (the signature ingredient of Chanel No. 19), and a sort of wet mossiness – a bit like the smell you get rootling around in the earth, tidying up the garden when spring's on its way, or walking into a florist's shop. We now live in a world of seriously complex fragrances, but this is worth checking out if you're looking for something with a simpler, more pared-down structure.

85 Prada Candy

Family: Gourmand
Launched: 2011
Creator: Daniela Roche-Andrier

Thierry Mugler's Angel was an 'olfactory shock' that carved out a whole new perfume category: gourmand, or 'edible' fragrances. Prada Candy has come along much later – but springing from one of the most lusted-after designer brands in the world, it attracted a whole new audience for gourmands. Quite rightly! If Angel is that entire dessert trolley, Prada Candy is 70 per cent dark chocolate. Straight from the bottle, it has a luminosity, while at the same time propelling a box of caramels at you. But then this swiftly mellows, becoming as cocooning and comforting as a pashmina. (For us, Prada Candy is very much autumn-winter, rather than spring-summer.) It's rich in sweet resins, including benzoin and tolu balsam, which are mysterious and enveloping, with amber adding a smoky darkness to the base. Candy is sensual, soft and powdery, with a cocktail of musks in the dry-down. 'It smells like skin, only better' is a comment that hits the mark for us. Oh, and this designer darling comes in a predictably stunning bottle, with its flash of shocking pink (but do be careful to position the nozzle or – like us – you may end up with an eyeful as well as a noseful).

86 Reiss Grey Flower

Family: Oriental
Launched: 2013
Creator: Azzi Glasser

The bottle looks like pure gold – and that's pretty much our verdict on what's inside the debut scent offering from fashion retailers Reiss. (The Duchess of Cambridge firmly put Reiss on the radar globally, 'papped' in many of their designs.) It's deep, it's woody, it's sensual – but rounded and snuggleable, too, with a real come-closer intimacy. Some intriguing ingredients: artemisia (wormwood), for its aromatic qualities, pimento berry for a touch of spice, cocoa leaf and 'amber crystals', alongside black jasmine, bay and lots of frankincense and patchouli. (If you like incense-based scents, you'll just adore this.) Grey Flower almost skips top notes and cuts straight to the chase: in perfumery, this is known as a 'linear' fragrance, which basically means that what you smell at first zoosh really is what you get. That 'linear' approach is becoming more popular in fragrance construction, because we live in an I-want-it-now world – even though we'd love everyone to take their time making their mind up about a scent, it doesn't always happen. Why the name? Inspiration was the soft grey tones of faded hydrangeas notwithstanding the fact they're actually unscented. Whatever: it's a treasure.

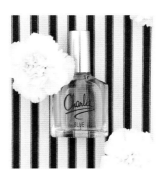

87 Revlon Charlie Blue

Family: Floral
Launched: 1973
Creator: Unattributed

We've included this for reasons of pure nostalgia– and because Charlie was such a landmark fragrance in its time, advertised by beautiful, smart-looking women striding out in trousers. (And even, in one ad, with a woman – shock, horror! – patting a besuited man's backside. 'Now the world belongs to Charlie!' said the voiceover.) For many women of 'un certain âge', this is time-warp stuff, created for the working woman who read *Cosmopolitan*, just waking up to the idea that she could have a sex life. (Charlie's working name was actually 'Cosmo'.) It was (and is) a very affordable way to get your hands on something that smells exactly like a classic French perfume: the usual citrussy introduction, a heart of hyacinth, jasmine, lily of the valley and carnation, a verging-on-chypre-y base of sandalwood, cedarwood, oakmoss, musk, cedar and vanilla, which dries down to a long-lasting woody, musky powderiness. Now for sure, Charlie isn't Guerlain, it's not Caron and it's definitely not Chanel but, nevertheless, Charlie has remained in production for over three decades. So put any perfume snobbery aside, take a sniff and decide: can all those Charlie-wearing women be wrong...?

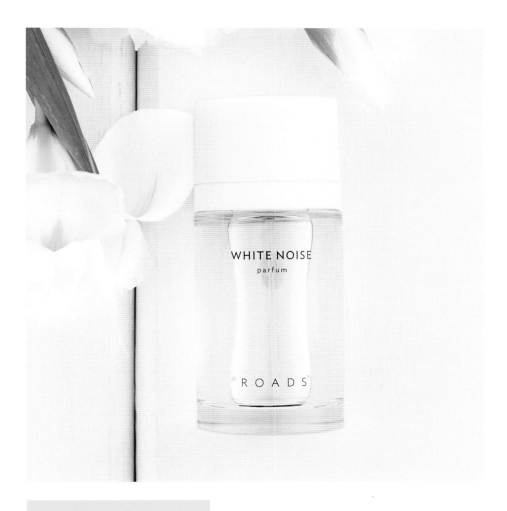

88 Roads White Noise

Family: Fresh **Launched:** 2014 **Creator:** Unattributed

It's not often (ever?) that a fragrance brand launches alongside arts projects, documentaries, feature films and books under the same umbrella – but Danielle Ryan's vision is to create a perfume brand influenced by all aspects of culture. Ambitious, yes (it's hard enough to get any budding fragrance business off the ground, without those complications) – but the real key for us is that the minimally-packaged collection of ten 'juices' themselves is completely beautiful, sometimes unusual but always wearable. (We first encountered them at Pitti Fragranze in Florence, one of two major annual perfume shows in Italy, showcased in a vast, all-white shipping container, with moving images flickering on the back wall.) Of the ten, we think this is likely to be the enduring bestseller: an almost 'abstract' composition that opens with a head-rush of aldehydes, lemon balm, green apple, mandarin and grapefruit. Then it mellows magically on the skin: soft iris, green violet leaf alongside those white flower pillars of jasmine and tuberose, with heliotrope: powdery, airy, pretty. Its lasting impression is quite woodsy, with sandalwood, cedarwood, amber and vanilla. We suggest you seek Roads out (at niche perfumeries), try them all – and see which floats to the surface for you.

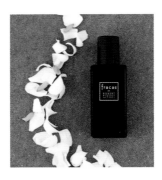

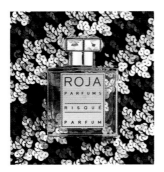

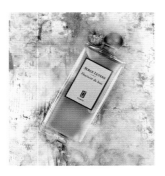

89 Robert Piguet Fracas

Family: Floral
Launched: 1948
Creator: Germaine Cellier

Piguet's tuberose-centric Fracas has had more facelifts than an octogenarian Hollywood Oscar-winner, but the fragrance community is generally agreed: it's back on form. And as Frederic Malle acknowledges: 'Every single person making a tuberose fragrance is trying to knock off the classic, which is Fracas.' Created by Germaine Cellier (who came up with Bandit, for the same house), it's sweet and strong and as in-your-face as a starlet's surgically inflated, Wonderbra-ed bosom: a tornado of white floral and green notes, in which tuberose wins out over gardenia, jasmine, lily of the valley, rose, neroli, iris and hyacinth. (And a sweeter-smelling bouquet than that it's hard to envision.) Light touches of bergamot and mandarin open Fracas up – and later on, under the throb of tuberose, the woody base positively purrs at you: cedar, vetiver and sandalwood. But basically, it's a big, big, tuberose. If you don't love that potent, exotic, sometimes almost medicinal floral ingredient, a bottle of Fracas will never find its way onto your dressing table. But as a landmark in fragrance history, make its acquaintance and try it on your skin – even if it turns out to be a one-night stand.

90 Roja Parfums Risqué

Family: Chypre
Launched: 2012
Creator: Roja Dove

Roja Dove spent many years at Guerlain before championing niche perfumers at his Harrods Haute Parfumerie boutique – and the fragrances he's launched under his signature line have a certain Guerlain-esque nostalgia, in quite a few cases, including this naughtily-named chypre treasure. (Alongside his own Roja Parfums line, Roja also offers a bespoke fragrance service; read more about this on page 96.) In Roja's own words, 'Risqué was inspired by the idea of ingredients so sexy that, if finely balanced, they have us on the verge of the forbidden.' Those sensual notes include the absolute classic pillars of a chypre: bergamot, oakmoss, labdanum, patchouli, alongside ambergris, vanilla, rose, ylang ylang, jasmine and narcotic hyacinth. It's got a definite leatheriness: imagine opening a well-cared-for vintage handbag, breathing in – and this is sort of what you'd get. (In a good way!) If you want to introduce your nose to the chypre family, there's almost nowhere better to start than Risqué. In its bling, diamanté-capped bottle, this is a nipped-in tailored suit of a fragrance: something you'd wear to lunch at The Ritz, or to listen to Verdi at La Scala, or to dine with a prince: sophisticated, sensual, superb.

91 Serge Lutens Féminité du Bois

Family: Woody **Launched:** 1992
Creator: Christopher Sheldrake

See-through, gauzy, hazy: Féminité du Bois is a mist, captured in a bottle. Violets – both the flower and the leaf – mix with dry woods and fruits to create something that always reminds us of a dream, half-remembered on waking but gone forever by the time we've turned the off alarm. In 1992, when the enigmatic make-up artist Serge Lutens launched his debut fragrance for Shiseido (the first in what is now a long line of extraordinary perfumes under his own name), it was a landmark scent: this much cedarwood didn't generally feature in feminine perfumery, even if it was softened by lush plummy notes, drizzled with honey and sprinkled with spices (think: cardamom, clove). More recently, Féminité du Bois has been reworked and moved into the so-successful Serge Lutens fragrance portfolio; some of the warm fruitiness has gone. But Féminité du Bois is still worth a spin. Though its sweetness has been toned down, this subtle scent is still dreamy: the spices and the other base notes (sandalwood and musk) quietly tiptoe in, making for an exquisitely well-rounded creaminess. With its fairy-like beauty, Féminité du Bois still doesn't smell like anything else we know. And we love it for that.

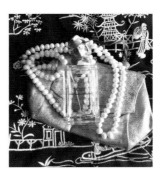

92 Sisley Eau du Soir

Family: Chypre
Launched: 1990
Creator: Jeannine Mongin

This fiercely green chypre is as sophisticated, as adult, as reach-for-your-tiara as a fragrance ever gets. It's probably physically impossible to wear it with jeans; it cries out for a night at Glyndebourne, or a very important black tie dinner party. Eau du Soir, from a skincare brand that ought to be way better known for its exquisite perfumes, is enigmatic, mysterious; you've got to have a ton of self-confidence to spritz this on to your pulse-points. Its overture is pure gin-and-tonic: dry, so dry, juniper-y with a twist of mandarin and citrus, a touch of apothecary's herb garden. But the true sophistication of Eau du Soir emerges with the heart notes: enveloping, cocooning, intriguing. It's dark, it's sultry, it's deep and mysterious. There's lilac (and the obligatory pillars of perfumery – jasmine and rose – albeit downplayed). The tiniest sweet breath of powder in there, too. And it has incredible staying power: this will be on your skin long, long after the curtain's gone down, the diva's picked up the roses strewn on the stage and the last autograph has been signed at the stage door. We can't help but think of it as the Rolls-Royce of chypres.

93 Thierry Mugler Alien

Family: Oriental **Launched:** 2005 **Creators:** Dominique Ropion and Laurent Bruyère

How do you follow a global success like Angel? It took Mugler more than a decade to have a go and as the designer acknowledged: 'Creating Alien was a huge challenge because now the whole world is watching'. The result certainly isn't as polarising as Angel (which we've grown to love), but coming from one of the most revered perfumers in the world – Dominique Ropion – it was never going to be bland. Mugler doesn't give much of the game away about what's in Alien, but you can be sure it's much more complex than 'top notes of jasmine sambac, middle notes of cashmere wood and base notes of white amber'. It's sweet, definitely vanilla-y, but a featherlight dusting rather than Angel's giant slug. There's some fleetingly sunny jasmine in there, but overwhelmingly we get dry, elegant woodsiness: it's all dark nightclubs and assignations and mystery. Lots of 'spins' on Alien now appear – that's how brands get great mileage out of a fragrance – which are instantly snapped up by devotees. But we like the original best, not least for its unique bottle – like a precious amulet straight out of *Game of Thrones*, if you ask us.

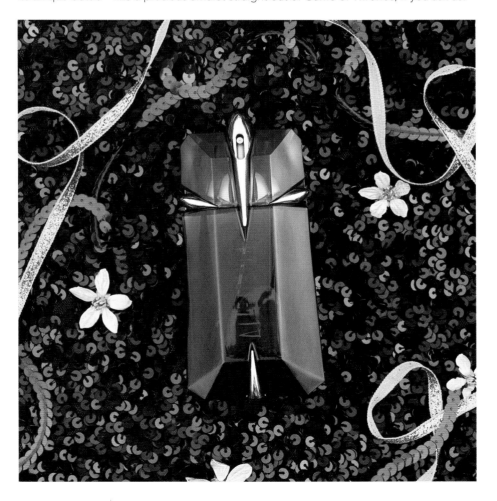

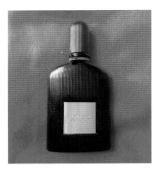

94 Tom Ford Black Orchid

Family: Oriental
Launched: 2006
Creators: David Apel and
Pierre Negrin

Black truffle? In a risotto, yes – but in a fragrance…? Trust Tom Ford to play tricks with our noses: in this complex, retro-elegant scent, it just adds another layer of dark, voluptuous fascination. The perfumista world was on tenterhooks to smell the former Gucci designer's first scent (and intrigued by his partnership with Estée Lauder Companies, which has turned out exceptionally well). Black Orchid didn't disappoint when launched, and still doesn't: an instant success, seriously 'femme fatale', it manages to be narcotic and fresh at the same time. Green, but with sweet gourmand qualities. After an invigorating first encounter with mandarin and bergamot, it segues into a seriously rich fusion of woody and vanilla notes: ylang ylang, black gardenia, jasmine and the eponymous 'Tom Ford Black Orchid' note (from one of the world's fragrant varieties), with a dry-down of amber, patchouli, incense, sandalwood, amber and vanilla. Not one for the office – never mind a meeting with your prospective in-laws – Black Orchid begs to be worn with a bias-cut white silk gown, a red lipstick, killer heels, and serious amounts of attitude. Up to the challenge?

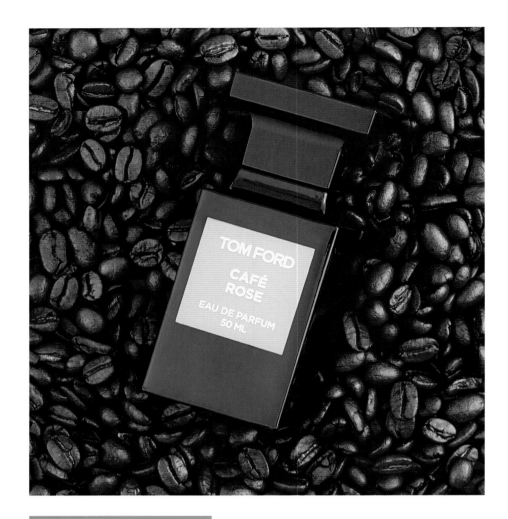

95 Tom Ford Café Rose

Family: Floriental **Launched:** 2012 **Creator:** Antoine Lie

All eyes – and all noses – have been trained on the Middle East in the past few years. The cradle of perfumery (the Arabian perfumers were mixing smoke and spices and woods with fairy dustings of rose milliennia ago), this area of the world has become hugely influential. Middle Easterners spend small (sometimes large) fortunes on fragrance, wearing as many as seven at once on their clothing and body, with money no object. The scent world has been clamouring for those dirhams and dinars by creating fragrances with more than a nod to perfume's Arabic heritage – but few have such global allure as this inky flacon of deliciousness. Sublimely rich and dew-drenched roses (Turkish, Bulgarian and May rose) make for a Turkish Delight sweetness. But a jolt of coffee – alongside a nose-tickling twist of black pepper – power this out of pretty-pretty floral territory into the realms of mystery, seduction, intrigue. Woven into an intricate tapestry of a base are breaths of sandalwood, patchouli, amber and incense, which swirl tantalisingly in and out. The whole Tom Ford collection begs to be explored but sit down with an espresso and take time to enjoy this.

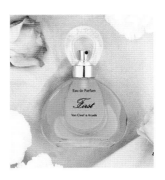

96 Van Cleef & Arpels First

Family: Floral
Launched: 1976
Creator: Jean-Claude Ellena

Nowadays every jeweller worth its diamonds has a fragrance – but this OTT floral helped pioneer the concept, back in the 1970s. It's all-dressed-up: we simply can't imagine wearing this beautifully rounded scent with jeans or for gardening; it's absolutely begging to be taken out for a candlelit dinner for two. First is a proper, grown-up and completely timeless perfume somewhat in the style of Chanel No. 5, with a similar sparkling wave of aldehydes at the beginning to instantly 'open up' the scent, inviting you to bury your nose in an exquisite bouquet of jasmine, Turkish rose, carnation, a touch of lily of the valley and hyacinth and the merest hint of sharp blackcurrant bud. The notes soften and become a little powdery on the body; it's as seamless and polished as a piece of marble, with every element melting into the next. As your evening wears on, a sort of honeyed quality emerges: amber and sandalwood, tonka bean and vetiver, adding further warmth. This is something worth exploring by someone at ease with their femininity, who loves the idea of finding a memorable 'signature scent' – but everyone needs to smell (and wear) this, in a lifetime. *Magnifique.*

97 Viktor & Rolf Flowerbomb

Family: Floral **Launched:** 2005 **Creators:** Olivier Polge, Carlos Benaïm and Domitille Bertier

Is it a floral? An Oriental? A gourmand? It's a sweet, seductive swirl of all three: incredibly pretty – and an instant global smash, despite the Dutch designers behind it not exactly being household names. It's not called 'bomb' for nothing: a couple of sprays are all you need to veil yourself in its cotton-candy deliciousness. (Lovers of Flowerbomb tell us how they just love coming across a scarf they've worn this with, and it's clung to.) Though caramel and vanilla don't feature on the 'official' list of ingredients, they're definitely in. And we're not surprised to discover that Flowerbomb is based on the 'gourmand patchouli' accord first introduced with Thierry Mugler's Angel, albeit in an altogether subtler package here. Flowerbomb manages (just) not to tip into over-sugariness, as the effervescent opening gives way to floral notes, flowing like honey one into another: jasmine sambac, freesia, rose, orchid, osmanthus – then amber, patchouli, musk. It's soft and fuzzy and a bit like snuggling under a cashmere blanket to watch your favourite ever film, with a mug of steaming hot chocolate in one hand, a glass of champagne on the coffee table and your best friend in the world curled up beside you.

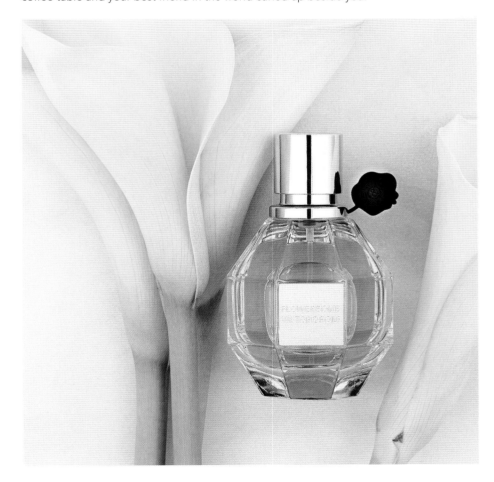

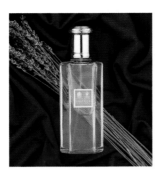

98 Yardley English Lavender

Family: Fresh
Launched: 1873
Creator: Unknown

A little bit of fragrance history in a bottle, this – and a scent that is almost certainly just as refreshing as when it launched, designed to delight a Victorian Britain in which single-note florals were 'trending' at the time. This is packed to the rafters with instantly uplifting and mind-soothing lavender – almost aromatherapeutic, we'd say, as well as a swift (shareable) pick-me-up in a bottle. The lavender smells real, very real, like rubbing the leaves and flowers through your fingers, although, as with all lavender notes, that doesn't hang around for long. (One devotee tells us she sprays it into her hair, and always gets compliments.) Although technically a single-note scent, it's way more complex than a simple distillation of 'lavender water'. There's bright bergamot and aromatic eucalyptus and rosemary in there, and lovely notes of geranium, clary sage and cedarwood in the heart. Smell your skin after a couple of hours, you might get little traces of tonka, musk and wet mossiness. Along with 4711 – another Cologne – this is one of the great 'fragrance steals', price-wise, that we know of. Splash and spray with abandon. Especially when energy or spirits are flagging, we suggest.

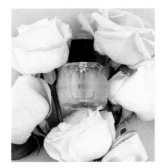

99 YSL Paris

Family: Floral
Launched: 1983
Creator: Sophia Grojsman

Paris, famously, is the world's most romantic city. And Sophia Grojsman's creation Paris is unquestionably pure romance, too. Delivered in a beautifully faceted, black-and-pink-stoppered bottle (designed by Pierre Dinand), it's happy, upbeat, with armfuls of roses, roses everywhere. The soft pastel 'juice' hints at Paris's femininity – but it's boldly feminine, rather than shyly girly; Paris, after all, was one of the iconic creations of the 1980s, when perfumes were constructed to announce a woman's presence. Nevertheless, it's floaty, breezy and sheer: prettily flirty, rather than overtly come-ravish-me. Sophia's influences for Paris include Guerlain's Après L'Ondée: 'I had the skeleton of a very creamy violet note. Then I worked on the rose to put with it…' So after a feather-light fruity-citrus introduction (bergamot, orange blossom), there's more than a smudge of violet in Paris: the roses scamper round and through that note, until its wonderful powdery softness rubs off on them. All the while, though, you can detect a cool greenness in the background: Paris is roses in a formal garden, hedged by evergreens, underpinned by a slight syrupiness. It's a love affair with roses you're after? *Voilà.*

100 YSL Rive Gauche

Family: Floral
Launched: 1970
Creator: Michel Hy

It's hard to imagine how groundbreaking this fragrance was: it was one of the first to tap into the seismic shift taking place between the sexes. While not targeted at 'bra-burners', Rive Gauche ('Left Bank', after Paris's artsier quarter) was daring, independent and as the translation of one ad from the French goes, 'Not for the unassuming woman'. You bought it for yourself; you didn't wait to be given it for a birthday. And you wore it with jeans, not a floaty frock. Rive Gauche is an 'abstract floral', in scent speak, but much greener than many florals. Even at first, you can make out wet, mossy notes, geranium and maybe a brief hint of smokiness. Then, just like a summer's morning, when the temperature climbs, those floral notes start to open, and warm up the fragrance, revealing rose, peach and lily of the valley, making for a soft powderiness. The woody dry-down (our favourite stage) takes a while to introduce itself: vetiver, sandalwood, oakmoss, musk and resins. (We could almost categorise this under chypres, actually: it bridges the two families.) What made Rive Gauche even more daring is that it came in a tin, not a bottle (still does). And it still dazzles, too, at fortysomething.

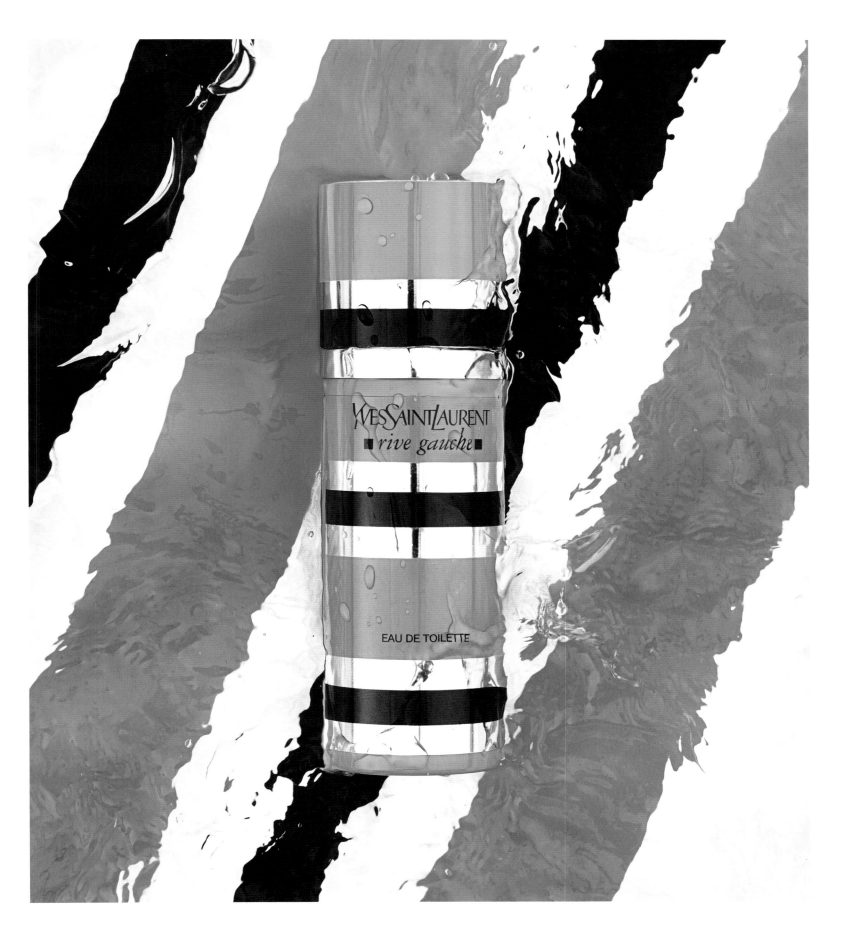

THE *men's* ROOM

There are almost – almost – as many male fragrances out there as there are women's, nowadays. (Of course, once upon a time, there was no division between the sexes when it came to perfumery; it was all 'shared'.) Some of the following scents are from well-known designer brands, others from more exclusive lines – but all are well worth a sniff

istock; marilyna/istock; rimglow/istock; dtimiraos/istock; Jim Parkin/Shutterstock

p58: Pol Barril

p59: Hajime Watanabe

p62–63: Vichly44/istock

p64 (left to right): LOOK Die Bildagentur der Fotografen GmbH/ Alamy; KUCO/Shutterstock; Jacky Parker/Alamy; niceartphoto/Alamy; Lidante/ Shuttsertock; Chris Hellier/Alamy; Angela Luchianiuc/ Shutterstock; Navè Orgad/Alamy; Christian Jung/Shutterstock

p67: Shutterstock/Gyorgy Barna

p70: Foster Curry

p72: Sam McKnight: Nick Knight; Maria Mosolova/Getty Images

p73 (left to right): Ursula Alter/Getty Images; Fumie Kobayashi/Getty Images; Chris Burrows/Getty Images; Jonathan Buckley

p74 (l to r): Visions/GAP Gardens; Boris SV/Getty Images; Jonathan Buckley; FhF Greenmedia/GAP Gardens; Jonathan Buckley

p76: The Advertising Archives

p77: The Advertising Archives

p78: The Advertising Archives

p79: The Advertising Archives

p83: Andreas von Einsiedel/Alamy

p85 (clockwise from top): Jessie Simmons; Studio des Fleurs; Atelier Cologne

p86: Editions de Parfums Frederic Malle; Grossmith

p87: Dominik Schulthess; Illuminum; Anaïs Biguine

p88: Jovoy; Elodie Farge & Charles Helleu; Derek Seaward

p89: Maison Francis Kurkdjian; Mary Greenwell; MEMO Paris

p90: Xavier Young; Roja Parfums; Tauer Perfumes

p91: Thirdman; Tom Daxon; Xerjoff

p93: Miller Harris Perfumer London

p94 (top to bottom): Camera Press London/J. Veysey; Miller Harris Perfumer London

p97: Foster Curry

p124 (right): Josephine Fairley

p137 (right): Josephine Fairley

p143 (left): Josephine Fairley

p144 (left): Josephine Fairley

p151 (left): Josephine Fairley

p158: Les Senteurs

p159 (clockwise from top): Christian Dietrich; MiN New York; Mark Hanauer

p160: Luckyscent, Inc.; Charlotte Mano; Jovoy

p161 (clockwise from top): Officina Profumo Farmaceutica di Santa Maria Novella; Anna Stowe Travel /Alamy; L'O Profumo

p163: wrangler/Shutterstock

We've had a huge amount of help and support with this book and so many thank-yous to say...

First, to The Perfume Society's amazing team: Ines Socarras, Alice Crocker, Alice Jones, Carson Parkin-Fairley, Rose Eastell and Lily de Kergeriest Gutierrez. Also to the 'home team' in Hastings: Amy Eason and David Edmunds, and to Paris Parkin-Fairley. This book may be dedicated to Craig Sams (along with Nick McKay) – but thanks for trudging down the stairs to sign for endless perfumes, Craig.

We'd like to thank our publisher Kyle Cathie, Julia Barder and our editor Vicky Orchard at Kyle Books, together with our wonderful agent Kay McCauley. (We still have hopes of finding the perfect scent for you, Kay.) Jenny Semple has designed a book more beautiful than our wildest imaginings, and Neal Grundy's pictures are stunning. Thanks to Kerrie Hess for illustrations that capture the joy of fragrance. Big thanks as ever for their ongoing support to Sue Peart and Catherine Fenton at YOU Magazine. And a big merci beaucoup to Sharon Whiting, The Perfume Bible's perfume-loving PR, and to Dowal Walker, The Perfume Society's PR agency.

Special thanks to the perfumers and creative directors who weave magical scents for us to enjoy, including Mandy Aftel, Roja Dove, Azzi Glasser, Sophia Grojsman, Lyn Harris, Francis Kurkdjian, Sarah McCartney, Jacques Polge and Christopher Sheldrake at Chanel, Linda Pilkington at Ormonde Jayne, Romano Ricci, Andy Tauer, Thierry Wasser at Guerlain. Special acknowledgment to Frederic Malle: not only a perfumer, but a man who helped to ignite the interest in perfumery which made this book so timely. (Thanks, too, to Pierre Dinand, and to Professor George Dodd.)

We also owe thanks to the perfume houses, beauty brands and fragrance distributors who have been so supportive of this project.

In alphabetical order (by perfume house/distributor): Stephane Euzen at Acqua di Parma. Lyndsay Fletcher at Aspects Beauty Company. Clive Christian. Amy Betsworth and Natalie Moon at Coty. Charlotte Mecklenburgh and Paula Smith at Elizabeth Arden. Jo Allison, Nathalie Everard and Penny Cross at Chanel. Clotilde Grange, Rebecca Filmer and Montasar Dumas at Dior. Chris Good at Estée Lauder and his fantastic team including

Meiissa Bancroft, Anna Bartle, Lizzie Brady, Trudi Collister, Jess de Bene, Claire Goodwin, Zoe Hardy, Melanie Jones, Lucie Seffens, Jay Squier, Amy Taylor and Pip Walsh. (Thanks, too, to Aerin Lauder.) Aisling Connaughton at Liz Earle – and of course, to Liz herself. Edward Bodenham at Floris. Howard Shaughnessy at Fragrance Factory. Our friend Kenneth Green and his Associates, including Nicola de Burlet, Fabien Callens and Linda Taylor. Rebecca Goswell and Mary Greenwell, creators of their own beautiful perfume houses. Kate Hudson, Jo Rash and Emily Field at Guerlain. Simon and Amanda Brooke at Grossmith. Keith Hamilton and Askala Geraghty at Illuminum. Clorinda di Tomasso and Morgan Ferrars at Intertrade, and Danielle Ryan of ROADS. François Hénin at Jovoy. Helen McTiffen at Lalique. Thierry Cheval, Emma Dawson, Charlotte Fielder, Charles de Montalevet, Amandine Ohayon, Kati Roberts and Sarah Williamson, at L'Oréal. Nick Gilbert at Penhaligon's. Jane McCorriston at Procter & Gamble. Simon Tuplin at Puig. Jack Cassidy at Roja Parfums. Shelley Smyth and her team at SAS & Company, including Elin Kikano, Sarah Tomlinson and Marion Leclerq. Sarah Duguid and Rebekah Watson at Sisley. Sheena Appadoo and Zoe Cook at The Body Shop. Laurent Delafon Jason Donovan at United Perfumes. Karen Cullen and Quentin Higham at Yardley.

To our PR agency friends, including Michelle Boon at Beautyseen. Rowley Weeks and Emma Elliott at Chalk PR. Fiona Dowal, Ali Pugh, Caroline Pugh, Jini Sanassay and Owen Walker at Dowal Walker. Rosa Sibaja at Frontrow PR. Genevieve Nikolopoulos and Carri Kilpatrick at Kilpatrick PR. Michael Donovan and Opinder Mehmi at Profile PR. Anna Zajicek at Purple PR. Katie Pearson at Smith & Monger. Julietta Dexter and Tom Konig Oppenheimer and their team at The Communications Store.

Thanks to Catherine Mitchell at International Flavors & Fragrances for help with the perfume portraits, to Linda Harman at Givaudan – and to Peter Norman and Linda Key at The Fragrance Foundation. To Claire Hawkesley and James Craven and their knowledgeable staff at Les Senteurs. To Sam McKnight for sharing his favourite scented flowers. And last but not least, Sarah Stacey, Jo's Beauty Bible co-author, for all her support and understanding during this time-consuming project...

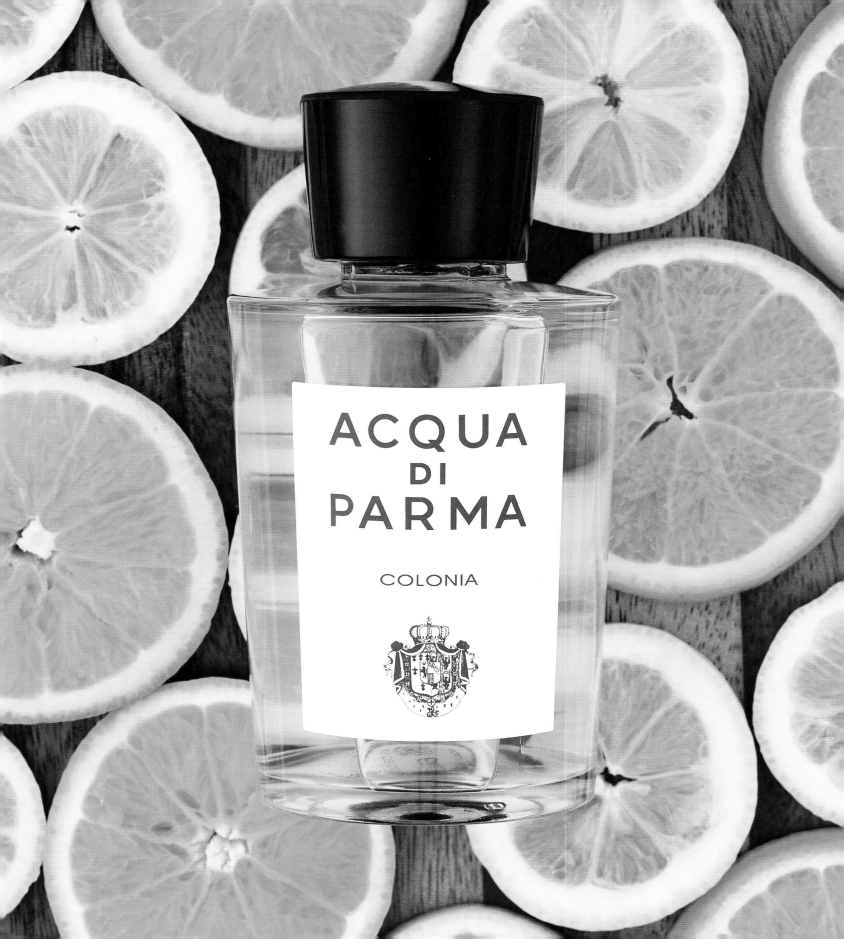

Acqua di Parma Colonia *(eau de Cologne)*

Family: Fresh
Launched: 1916
Creator: Unattributed

Colonia originally made its debut in 1916 but this classic Cologne is wearing so, so well. It'll wake you up in the morning faster than a double espresso: a splash of sharp citrussy notes of bitter orange, lemon and Sicilian bergamot. Then as the bracing top notes fade, it's time for the herbal green elements – rosemary, clary sage, lavender, verbena – to take over. This aromatic heart is fairly long-lasting, softened just a little by a powdery dusting of Bulgarian rose and iris, rounding its crisp edges. It's definitely got much more going on than most eaux, yet still smells revivingly clean and fresh throughout. As one reviewer put it, 'This is my go-to scent when I just want to smell nice – not showy, avant-garde or in your face.' (There are plenty of other scents for that.) It's easy to wear, easy to love (and dead easy to 'borrow' from him). The sunshine yellow outer box is a classic, too, with its simple lettering and the coat of arms of Parma, Italy. Too good to throw away, we think it makes a great desk accessory – maybe one of the sexiest paperclip or pencil holders ever.

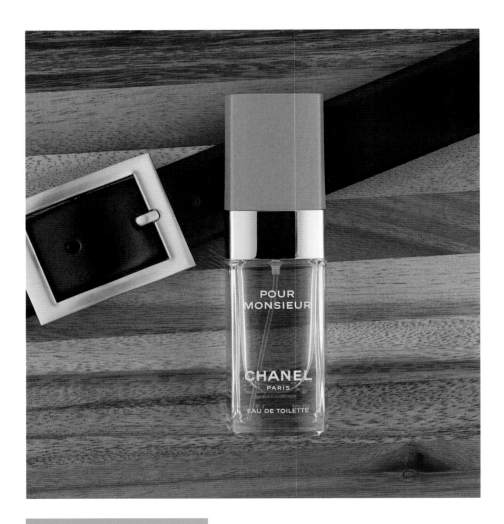

Chanel Pour Monsieur

Family: Fougère **Launched:** 1955 **Creator:** Henri Robert

Pour Monsieur also has all the freshness of a traditional Cologne, and, actually, these haven't strayed far from the original centuries-old formulation – heavy on the refreshing citrus notes (think: neroli, petitgrain, lemon), and generally with some lavender woven in. But underneath the just-stepped-from-the-shower freshness of Pour Monsieur is an extra layer of intrigue: a little dusting of ginger and cardamom spiciness (definitely staying this side of chai, however). What's really interesting is that, after a while on the skin, it mellows and softens as the base layer of pencil-case-y cedarwood, oakmoss and damp, earthy vetiver emerge. Eventually, you get a lovely, lingering – but very subtle – powderiness, (which makes this very 'shareable' by women who don't like their scents too frou-frou). Pour Monsieur was created by Henri Robert – the same in-house 'nose' who brought us Chanel No. 19 – in the Mad Men era of the mid-1950s, when men (or at least, those who weren't wearing bike leathers and listening to Elvis) aspired to good grooming and good manners. It not only ticks both those boxes, but that's exactly how it was originally marketed, as a real gentleman's fragrance. Still easy-to-wear, still easy-to-love today.

Davidoff Cool Water

Family: Fresh **Launched:** 1988 **Creator:** Pierre Bourdon

Fresh. Sporty. Sexy. Advertised by a half-naked man against a background of azure sea or crashing surf. This entire, vast fragrance category has been influenced by Davidoff Cool Water, which smells as unlike a cigar as anything we've ever had wafted under our nostrils. Cigars…? Why, yes: Zino Davidoff was a purveyor of the highest-quality Cuban cigars (and once taught Jo, co-author of this book, how to smoke one, for a journalistic assignment!). The blockbuster success of this so-fresh, easy-sea-breezy scent, though, eclipses any tobacco-baron reputation Davidoff may have had: it's a true fragrance icon, as splashable today as it was in the 1980s when it powered onto the perfumed radar. There's a good reason scent critic Luca Turin awarded it 'five stars': Cool Water is a wonderful, poised balance of aromatic notes – lavender, coriander, rosemary, peppermint (and we get hints of fresh-cut grass) – on a dead-sexy, come-and-get-it base of musk, cedar, sandalwood, amber and oakmoss, which leave sensual, damp moss trails on the skin. In between? If you sniff very carefully, you might get little wafts of geranium. We've hardly ever met a man who – secretly or loudly-and-proudly – doesn't rather love this classic. Which is quite a feat.

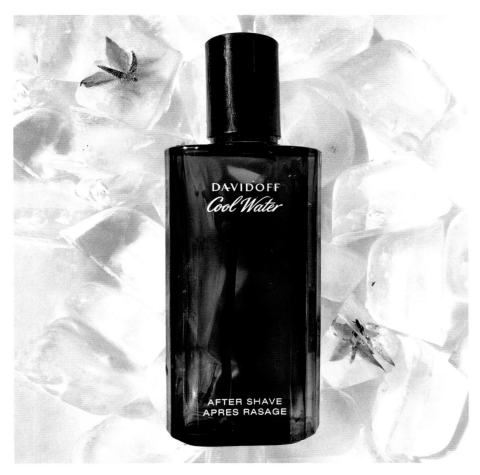

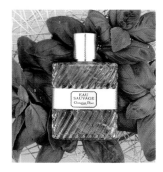

Dior Eau Sauvage

Family: Fresh
Launched: 1966
Creator: Edmond Roudnitska

One lemon-sherbet-y blast of this and we're taken straight back to a time when we wore this ourselves. (And so did many women: the hip flask-inspired bottle sits equally well on either side of the bathroom shelf – His or Hers.) Eau Sauvage is a Cologne with the lemon ramped up, along with petitgrain, which somehow makes it even lemonier, adding a green edge. Aromatic rosemary and basil also feature, and lots of vetiver in the base, along with the classic chypre staple oakmoss, and maybe a touch of musk, too. It was also one of the fragrances to pioneer the use of a synthetic called hedione, which is a bit jasmine-y, a little bit aquatic – but overall it's very pared-down, the product of Edmond Roudnitska's desire to simplify his approach to perfumery. (He also created Diorissimo.) But less is very definitely more, here: it's still effortlessly fresh, clean and sexy. Part of the joy of this fragrance, right from the first time we tried it, was re-spraying it and re-spraying it all over again. (Especially at 4pm, when it's better than even the strongest cup of black tea for reviving flagging energy and mood.)

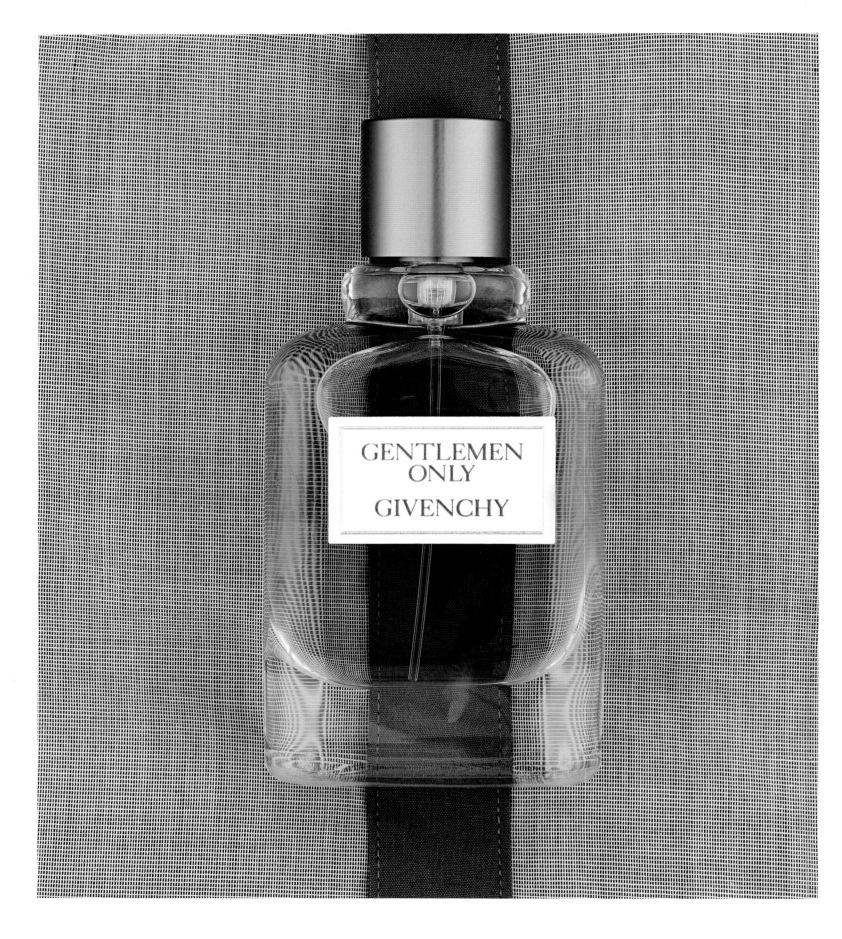

Givenchy Gentleman Only

Family: Woody
Launched: 2013
Creator: Unattributed

Few men have embodied elegance like Hubert de Givenchy (who we once had the pleasure of meeting): tall, immaculate, super-stylish, the man who dressed film star legends like Audrey Hepburn, who rarely wore any other designer. It was in Hubert de Givenchy's day, presiding over his couture house, that the original Givenchy Gentleman was created – and became male fragrance legend, with its big, blatant patchouli note, earthy and primal. We love it – but we concede that GG may not play with a younger audience: the equivalent of wearing a starched shirt to the office on dress-down Friday. The iconic Givenchy Gentleman is still the 'inspiration' for this new version, however: a woody aromatic scent with uplifting top notes of mandarin and pink pepper, touches of tarry birch at its heart, on a classically woody base of cedar, patchouli, vetiver. Most definitely worthy of the label 'a new classic', it's actually quite understated – the embodiment of good taste, in a bottle. Speaking of the bottle, it's satisfyingly chunky – much too stylish to hide in the bathroom cupboard. (And do give Givenchy Gentleman itself a sniff, too. Preferably on the neck of somone you're mad for.)

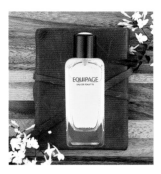

Hermès Equipage

Family: Fougère
Launched: 1970
Creator: Guy Robert

This masterpiece was the very first male fragrance from luxury leather house Hermès and it's still the embodiment of masculine elegance. But we believe it's worth discovering by a younger generation than the fathers and grandfathers who've grown older wearing this as their refined, understated signature, as an antidote to footballers' scents, rappers' scents and countless 'celeb' launches. Contrastingly aromatic and spicy, it's lively with notes of marjoram, hyssop, tarragon and cinnamon, and the cloviness of carnation. But there's a subtle floral quality to Equipage (from teeny-tiny puffs of jasmine, lily of the valley) that makes it perfectly shareable: we're all for women dabbing on something a bit more virile, occasionally. You can't especially identify the vetiver, the patchouli, the amber or the vanilla-esque tonka bean in the base of Equipage: it's all so seamless. But they give a leathery, earthy smokiness that is rich, rich, rich. Still, definitely 'old money', rather than nouveau riche, this one. And we love this online comment from one Equipage-lover, in a Fragrantica fragrance forum: 'For "men" – so wait until you're at least in your thirties, have a job, a house, a car – not necessarily a wife yet: this will help!'

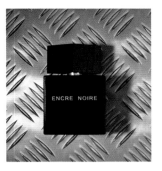

Lalique Encre Noir

Family: Woody
Launched: 2006
Creator: Nathalie Lorson

In our humble opinion, one of the sexiest smells a man can wear is vetiver: dark, mysterious, earthy, woody. It's an ingredient that consistently inspires perfumers, who can put a fresh spin on it, or play up vetiver's inherent mystery, accenting darker and more smokily smouldering facets. And this creation – from the celebrated glass manufacturer – has gone over to the dark side, in absolutely the best way. It's a gold standard vetiver, with a scrunch of black pepper and a 'bonfire moment', after the fleeting, fresh top notes have vanished. It's elegant and refined and would make any man who wore it seem not just intriguing, but worth getting much closer to – if only so that you can sniff his neck. Once there, you might be able to make out notes of cypress, Bourbon vetiver (from the isle of Réunion, off Madagascar – also famous for its vanilla), and Haitian vetiver, too. (Like wine, perfume ingredients are affected by 'terroir': the same ingredient, harvested from different parts of the world, may have a different character.) In the long-lasting base, soft cedarish woods and musks swirl together for hours. But one sniff and we're lost, actually. And darn, the ink-black bottle's fab.

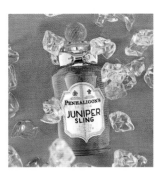

Penhaligon's Juniper Sling

Family: Woody
Launched: 2011
Creator: Olivier Cresp

Gin and tonic, anyone? First spritz from this bow-tied bottle, and you'll definitely be hoping the sun will soon be over the yardarm, making it time to reach for the London Dry Gin that inspired this innovative scent. It's fresh and original and we absolutely love it: a playful creation from Olivier Cresp, who's A Very Big Name in the 'nose' world. A generous slug of juniper has been blended with wonderfully complementary aromatic and spicy notes: green and almost musky angelica, a generous grind of black pepper, a touch of cinnamon and cardamom, then ever-so-slightly sweetened with a touch of iris. Juniper Sling is thirst-quenchingly fresh and outdoorsy until the warmer, nuzzleable base notes emerge: earthy vetiver, soft amber – and a touch more sweetness from a sugar note. (We still get juniper right through till the last, fading whiff, though.) It's not incredibly long-lasting – more akin to a Cologne – but for men who don't want to smell like everyone else, a very stylish choice. (Eminently shareable, too.) Gorgeous bottle – inside a silver-and-green box that's almost too handsome to throw away.

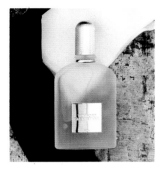

Tom Ford Grey Vetiver

Family: Woody
Launched: 2009
Creator: Unattributed

Vetiver turns out to be a very versatile fragrance ingredient. It can have a dark-and-smouldering spin put on it, or be lightened and freshened, making it smell more like the deep-rooted grass that it is. Encre Noir (see page 153) falls into the first category, but this is a breezy, airy vetiver, which gets off to a throw-open-the-windows sunny start: a blast of grapefruit, orange flower, hints of aromatic sage. It has a soft heart, buttered-up by iris – and lavender, we think, because this is almost classically 'Cologne-y' at times. As sure-footed as almost every Tom Ford we've ever smelled, Grey Vetiver mellows to a very classic spicy-woody-smoky masculine base, that signature vetiver rubbing along nicely with light touches of vanilla-y toasted tonka (as well as vanilla itself), oakmoss, amber woods, and touches of black pepper. This scent is crisp, smart and sharp (in the well-dressed sense of the word), easy to wear in a work environment or as a swiftly reviving spritz, after a tough day. We can't recommend too highly that a man should explore the vetiver world – and as one commentator put it, 'Grey Vetiver would be a great place to start your vetiver education.'

Yohji Homme

Family: Woody
Launched: 1999
Creator: Jean-Michel Duriez

Men all over the world went into mourning when the original Yohji Homme (from the Japanese designer Mr Yamamoto) was discontinued. The good news is that this quirky, swimming-against-the-tide 'cult' men's scent is back, reinterpreted by 'nose' Olivier Pescheux. And very interesting – yet wearable – it is, too. Fresh notes and spices are combined incredibly successfully: servings of coffee, mocha and rum jostle for space in the tall, sleek cylindrical glass bottle, with more traditional men's ingredients such as cedarwood, bergamot, sage, lavender, juniper, plus a spicy dusting of cardamom. Leather, musk and patchouli make themselves known in the base, and, in our experience, it lasts for hours on the skin, without intruding rudely into anyone's workspace (although it's equally appropriate for casual weekends and one perfume blogger described it as 'the closest thing to bottled rock 'n' roll I have yet encountered.') When Yohji Homme was first released, the designer called it 'a scent that follows the funny off-track and avant-garde image of my fashion'. Something for a confident man who doesn't need to dress – or smell – like anyone else, but is comfortable in his own rather attractive skin.

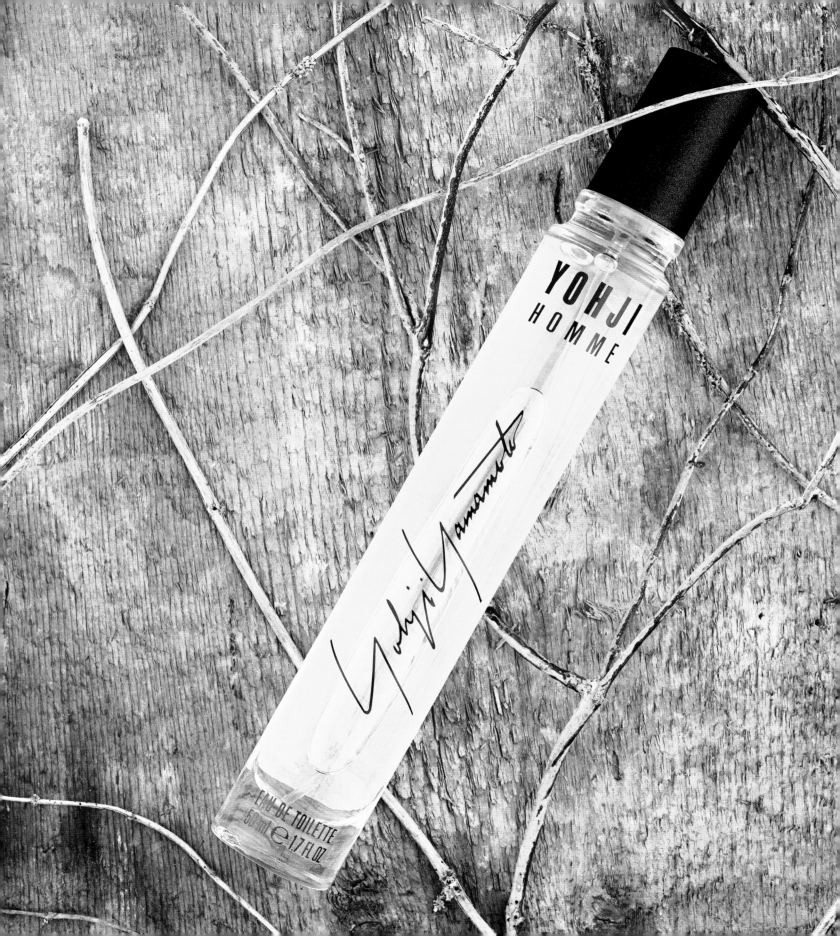

" You see, perfume awakens thought

Victor Hugo

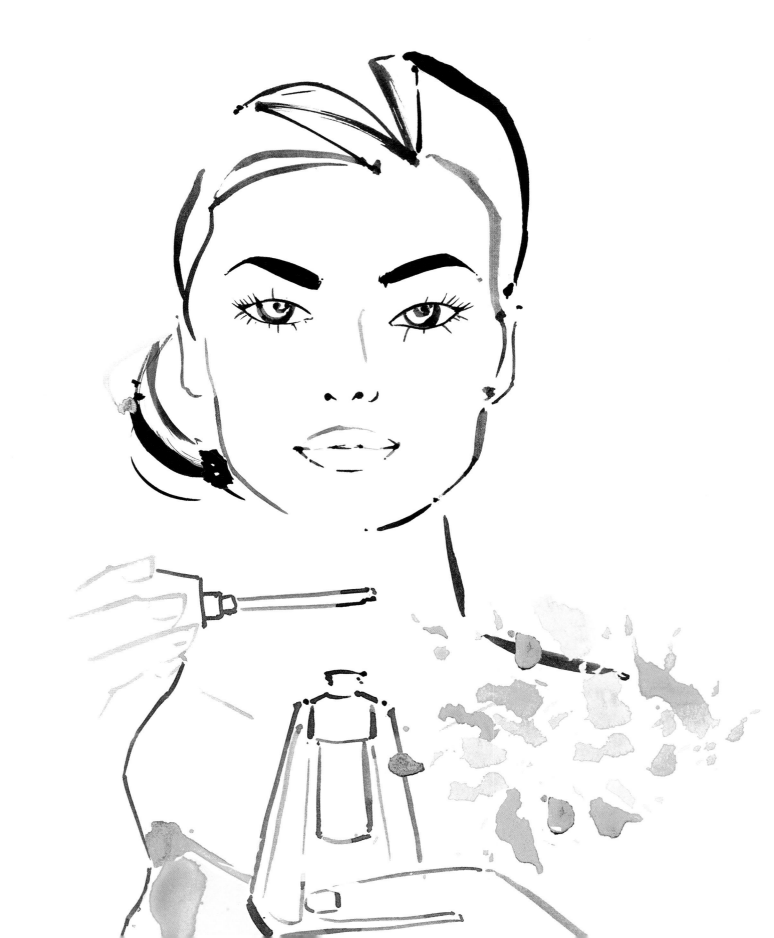

(SOME OF)
THE BEST
perfume shops
IN THE WORLD

We could write an entire, global guide to fragrance shopping. (If you ask nicely enough, perhaps we will…!) For us, sniffing out new smells and scents is part of the joy of travel: we just love to discover new stores and small boutiques – and even souks – to shop in, or simply to waft new and different fragrances under our noses and deepen our appreciation. Here are a few highlights on our global perfume-shopping map…

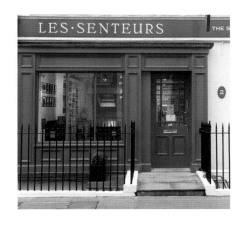

Les Senteurs (London, UK) The Hawksley family has been showcasing independent perfumery brands for over 30 years, first in Pimlico and now also just north of Mayfair, where second-generation perfume-lover Claire presides over a team of incredibly knowledgeable staff. Generous sampling (they'd always rather you took something away and allowed it to grow on you, rather than making a snappy mistake) and a welcoming vibe make this shop a joy to visit and linger in as you explore dozens of brands from Frederic Malle to Serge Lutens, By Kilian, Ireland's Cloon Keen Atelier, 4160 Tuesdays, Caron, etc.
71 Elizabeth Street, Belgravia, London SW1W 9PJ
Tel: 00 44 (0)20 7730 2322
www.lessenteurs.com

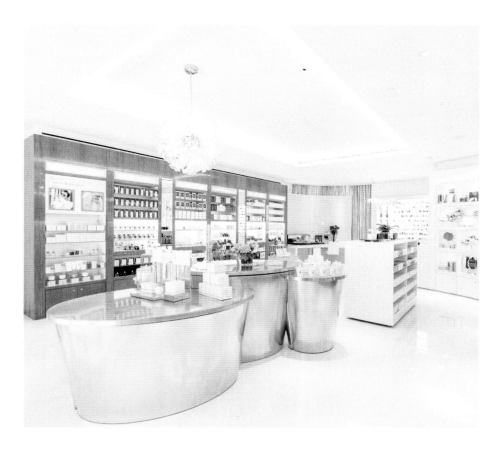

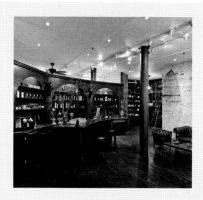

MiN NY (New York, USA) Our two absolute favourite New York perfume destinations are both in SoHo. (NB There's also a stunning fragrance department in the basement of Bergdorf Goodman.) This store has incredibly highly trained staff, a really interesting portfolio of niche fragrances, a 'men's zone' – and a cocktail bar, if you need refreshment while you shop. It's a put-your-feet-up-on-the-ever-so-slightly-scuffed-sofa type of place, accessorised by antiques – and we feel right at home.
117 Crosby Street, New York, NY10012 (between East Houston and Prince)
Tel: 00 1 212 206 6366
www.min.com

Osswald (New York, USA) Just the polar opposite to MiN NY's dark, clubby feel (right), Osswald is very bright, white and almost clinical (probably a nod to its Swiss heritage). But it has a stunning selection of independent perfumes, including Francis Kurkdjian, Amouage, Clive Christian and Roja Parfums.
311 West Broadway, New York, NY 10013 (between Canal and Grand)
Tel: 00 1 212 625 3111
www.osswaldnyc.com

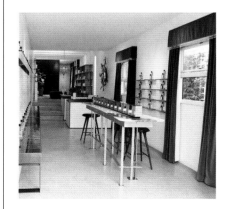

Strange Invisible Perfumes (Los Angeles, USA) We have to include the Strange Invisible Perfumes boutique on cool-and-groovy Abbot Kinney Boulevard; most of the shops listed in this chapter offer a wide selection of brands, but this one is entirely devoted to perfumer Alexandra Balahoutis's collection of purely organic, wild-crafted, biodynamic and 'hydro-distilled' fragrances, with names such as Fair Verona, Epic Gardenia, Prima Ballerina and Dimanche. If you can possibly stretch to it, treat yourself to the 'Perfume Minibar': a beautiful box of 12 different samples. Not cheap, but seriously swoon-worthy.
1138 Abbot Kinney Boulevard, Venice, CA 90291 Tel: 00 1 310 314 1505
www.siperfumes.com

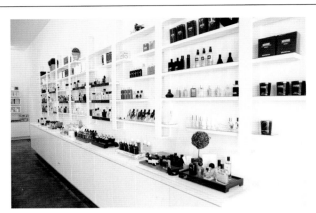

Scent Bar (Los Angeles, USA) This is the 'bricks-and-mortar' incarnation of www.luckyscent.com, which is the US's best-known retailer of hard-to-find perfume brands. This airy Beverly Boulevard store was created to 'offer the intimacy of a wine bar without the formality' (it does indeed have a bar-like design), inviting you to sit and discover creations from Testa Maura, Serge Lutens, Agonist, Byredo, Andrea Maack, Grossmith… A real A–Z of glorious 'finds', with a classically laid-back Californian welcome.
7405 Beverly Boulevard, Los Angeles, CA 90036
Tel: 00 1 323 782 8300
www.luckyscent.com

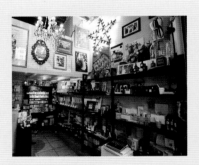

Marie-Antoinette (Paris, France) Barely bigger than a shoebox, Marie-Antoinette's passionate owner and 'curator' manages to shoehorn dozens of independent brands into this Marais-based perfumery with great style, making it feel like the perfume equivalent of a delicious box of chocolates. Find Vero Profumo, Parfums d'Orsay, Houbigant, Ineke and more, more, more. An utter delight and a treat. (But do double-check the address before heading there, as owner Antonio de Figueiredo tells us he's searching for new – and possibly larger! – premises.)
Place du marché Sainte Catherine, 5 rue d'Ormesson, 75004 Paris, France Tel: 00 33 1 42 71 25 07
www.marieantoinetteparis.fr

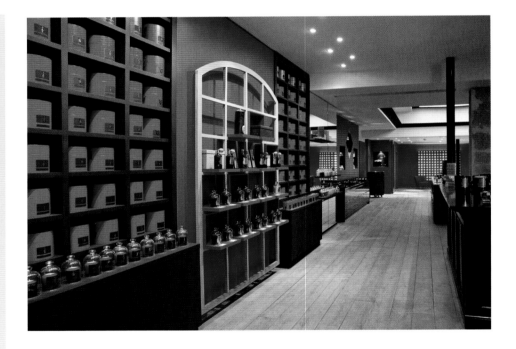

Jovoy (Paris, France) If you have only one day in Paris and want to experience the absolute widest possible selection of niche perfumes, head straight here. In a setting of chic Chinese red walls and reclaimed shop furniture from past eras (not to mention some rather spiffy 1950s sofas and chairs at the rear of the shop), owner François Hénin has brought together some of the most bewitching and beguiling independent perfume lines in the world, including Puredistance, Neela Vermeire, Nasomatto, Parfums de Marly: a 'Who's Who' of everything that's interesting in perfumery at any given moment in time.
4 Rue de Castiglione, 75001 Paris, France Tel: 0 33 1 40 20 06 19
www.jovoyparis.com

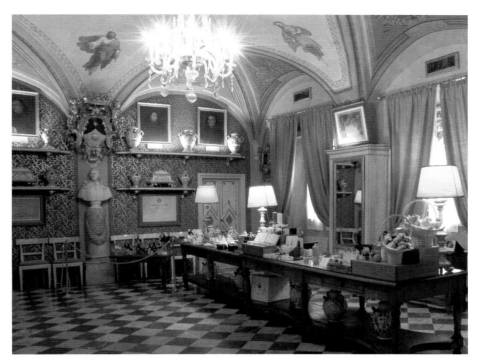

Farmaceutica di Santa Maria Novella (Florence, Italy) There's been a pharmacy here since 1612 and in the back of this extraordinary, almost church-like store (which leads into a monastery) there is still a dispensary handing out potions and tonics. There are now dozens of fragrances in Santa Maria Novella's portfolio, many of them Colognes, including fragrances such as Tuberosa, Verbena and Vetiver – but the most famous and sought-after is probably Melograno (pomegranate). Don't leave without treating yourself to a box of the spicy potpourri, which will scent a room for years.
Via della Scala 16, 50123 Firenze, Italy Tel: 00 39 055 216276
www.smnovella.it

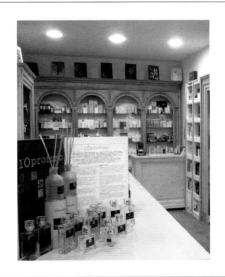

L'O Profumo (Florence, Italy) One of the most extraordinarily comprehensive fragrance offerings we've ever stumbled upon on our travels, in a long, slim shop on an undistinguished street in Florence. Creed, Heeley, État Libre d'Orange, Jardins d'Écrivains, Tauer, Mark Buxton, Keiko Mecheri, Olfactive Studio – oh, over 60 brands altogether. You could spend an entire day here without getting bored (although your nose might get a tad weary).
Via Pietrapiana 44, 50121 Firenze, Italy Tel: 00 39 055 2639657
www.loprofumo.com

The Dubai Perfume Souk
(Dubai, UAE) Man, there are some stinkers here – but if you really want to get your nostrils around Arabian perfume culture and, in particular, its love affair with intense, love-them-or-hate-them ingredients such as oudh and frankincense, wander through the streets of this souk and spend an hour or two visiting the various stores, where shopkeepers can help you select something that's to your taste among their attars and essences. Be prepared to haggle. The large department stores at the various Dubai malls also carry a huge range of international fragrances, satisfying a demand in a country where it's not unusual to wear up to seven fragrances at a time. (Yes, really!)
Sikkat al Khail Road, Deira (just east of the Gold Souk)

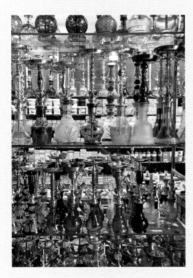

PS We're always on the hunt for fabulous new fragrance boutiques to visit, so if you have a favourite do email us at: email info@perfumesociety.org. We'd love to hear from you.

perfume and the
BLOGOSPHERE

Thanks entirely to the internet, something wonderful has happened in the past few years to open people's eyes – and our minds (never mind our nostrils) – to the extraordinary wealth of perfumes out there

'The bloggers', as they're known, are independent perfume critics who generally don't make a living out of perfume reviewing – not when they first start, anyway – but who do it for pure passion. They're based all over the world: the UK, America, Australia, Greece (most write in English). We follow many of them ourselves as part of an ongoing mission to discover new creators and brands – and be reminded of old favourites, which have become neglected in our quest to try everything new and exciting that crosses our desks.

Some of the most gifted perfume writers in the world can be read and followed on the web entirely for free. We keep these bookmarked and heartily recommend

you read what they have to say as part of your ongoing 'perfume education' – because as with wine, art or literature, the more you soak up about a subject, the deeper your knowledge becomes, the more pleasure you get out of it.

These blogs are also great for keeping your finger on the pulse – or should it be pulse-point? – of what's happening on the scent front.

Persolaise Dariush Alavi has justly won Jasmine Awards (the perfume industry's 'literary Oscars') for his writing; he's since written a book about niche perfumery, *Le Snob: Perfume*. Dariush reviews when inspiration strikes and does occasional interviews with perfumers, too. We think

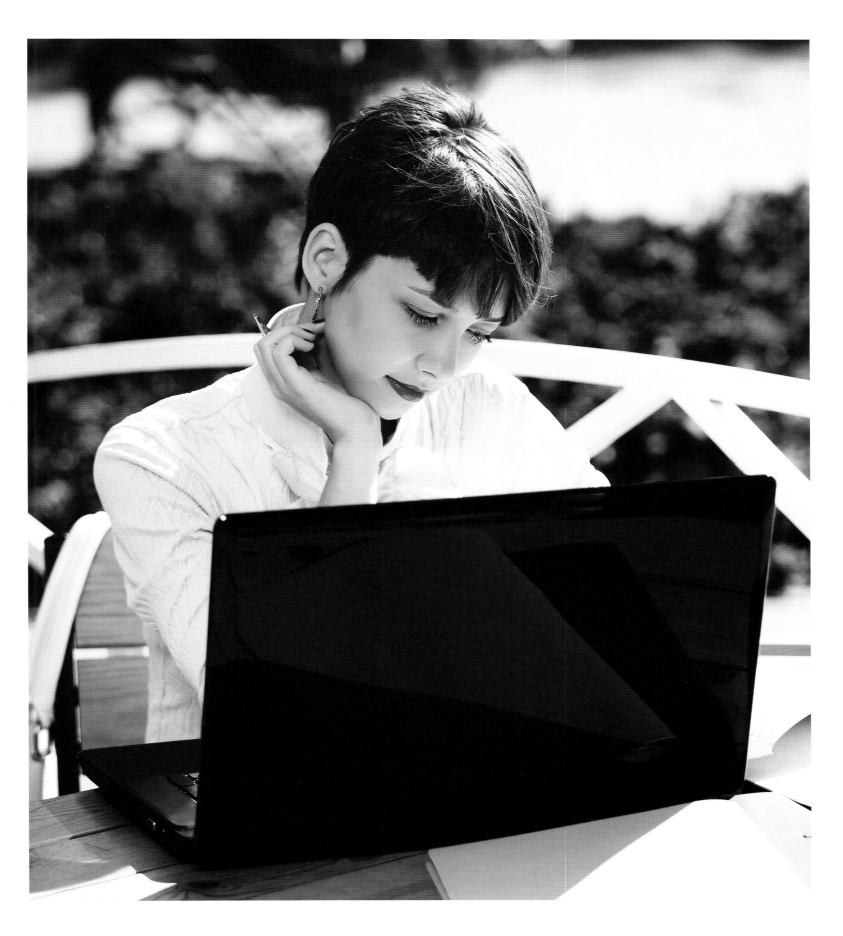

his writing is among the best out there and follow it fairly slavishly. www.persolaise.blogspot.co.uk

Katie Puckrik Smells
American-born, British-based Katie offers something different: because of her background as a TV presenter, this self-confessed 'thrill-seeker when it comes to scent' has her own YouTube channel of perfume reviews. And unlike so many video reviews on YouTube, these are really informative and worth watching, brilliantly bringing scents to life. Don't bother with the rest: save yourself a lot of time and just tune into Katie.
www.katiepuckriksmells.com

The Non-Blonde
As New Jersey-based Gaia Fishler puts it, 'I try stuff so you don't have to.' (Which also includes beauty products, as well as fragrances.) As well as individual perfume reviews, Gaia's really great at writing longer features that group similar scents together on a theme: rose, iris, smoky, citrus, amber, etc.
www.thenonblonde.com

Now Smell This
An absolutely brilliant, all-embracing blog, which has grown into a mini-website, really, showcasing great reviews and features; it's also one of the best sites for staying on top of new and upcoming releases. The site's editor, Robin, is 'an avid perfume fan living in a small town in Pennsylvania, far from the nearest perfume store'.
www.nstperfume.com

Perfume-Smellin' Things
If you can manage not to be distracted by the flashing ads in the margins, there's some really good stuff here: excellent reviews (mostly of niche and 'cult' scents) from a select band of bloggers. Definitely worth a dip.
www.perfumesmellinthings.blogspot.co.uk

Savvily, editors have scanned the blogosphere and signed up some of the most expressive writers for print

Perfume Posse
The bloggers at this US-based site have been hard at work reviewing since 2005 (edited by Patty White), so there's a ton of stuff on this site, which was voted one of the 'Best Perfume Blogs' by the Huffington Post for its conversational, witty style. There are good, basic introductions to discovering niche perfumery, pointing you in the direction of plenty of interesting stuff to smell, with comprehensive guides to the 'best' perfumes in specific categories (vetiver, vanilla, rose, etc.).
www.perfumeposse.com

Bois de Jasmin
One of our favourites, so beautifully written and yet packed with lots of practical info on the world of perfume, from how it's made to how to choose and wear it. Victoria Frolova, based in New York and Brussels, also contributes to the *Financial Times* and *Perfumer & Flavorist* magazines. (Savvily, editors have scanned the blogosphere and signed up some of the most expressive writers for print.)
www.boisdejasmin.com

Perfume Shrine
Editor Elena Vosnaki – a fragrance historian and writer based in Greece – has incredible depth of knowledge about ingredients, trends and history (no surprise there) and combines them with her musings about sensual pleasures and the art of perfumery. Literally thousands of postings; if you're not careful you could lose weeks of your life here.
www.perfumeshrine.blogspot.com

Grain de Musc
Denyse Beaulieu is a writer and translator based in Paris, who's gone on to write a book about her real-life passion for fragrance and where it's led her: *The Perfume Lover: A Personal History of Scent*, which also traces the creation of a real-life perfume created by 'nose' Bertrand Duchaufour for L'Artisan Parfumeur, Sevilla à l'Aube. Get over the so-basic design: there's lots

to explore here, including insightful interviews with many of the globally renowned 'noses' based in Denyse's home town.
www.graindemusc.blogspot.com

The Scented Salamander Packed, packed, packed with fragrance news and reviews (the 'Perfume Shorts' are great bite-sized temptations), this was one of the pioneering blogs so its archive is immense. Scented Salamander is written by Chantal-Hélène Wagner, a gifted writer with a PhD in Anthropology and Oriental Studies – so her writing's very in-depth and often looks at fragrance in a 'wider context'.
www.mimifroufrou.com

Cafleurebon (Say it: 'sah-fleur-bohn'.) A beautifully-written blog with almost daily postings (though you slightly have to shut your eyes to the flashing ads right, left and centre…). Cafleurebon has some terrific in-depth articles on ingredients, interviews with perfumers and reviews of (mostly niche) perfumes both new and old; editor-in-chief is beauty and scent journalist Michelyn Camen.
www.cafleurebon.com

Candy Perfume Boy London-based Thomas (who works in HR but is a gifted 'self-proclaimed perfume addict') has scooped a coveted Jasmine Award for his blog-writing: this is an enchanting, very personal site, with – alongside a torrent of reviews – some great in-depth features on different fragrance ingredients and the many and various ways perfumers have chosen to showcase them. (It was his article 'The Candy Perfume Boy's Guide to Violet', which scooped the prize.)
www.thecandyperfumeboy.com

If you fancy yourself as a 'perfume critic' (and it seems that gazillions do), there are two incredibly comprehensive, information-packed websites that encourage threads of comments on

The Perfume Society is an actual real-life community – the first perfume appreciation society in the world

thousands of fragrances:
www.basenotes.com and
www.fragrantica.com

And can we just declare an interest, here…? The Perfume Society website (www.perfumesociety.org) and The Scent Critic are our own projects. Much more than just a website, The Perfume Society is an actual real-life community – the first perfume appreciation society in the world – which perfume lovers can join, with events, meet-ups and sampling opportunities; the website itself is updated constantly with perfume news (and we produce our own online magazine for subscribers, The Scented Letter). In addition, Jo writes occasional reviews of fragrances that have rocked her boat on www.thescentcritic.com – though less often now The Perfume Society is basically a full-time mission.

The internet, as you've probably realised, is also a bit like a game of tennis-elbow-foot: one thing rapidly leads to another as you follow links. Most good perfume blogs have 'blogrolls': lists of other recommended sites. Start with those above – and then follow where your mouse leads. Just don't blame us if you never make it back from Narnia.

TIP

Applying fragrance to your clothes is a lovely way to wear it – but be cautious…

Spritz a piece of kitchen roll or a tissue with the fragrance and check that it doesn't stain or mark the fabric: amber-coloured fragrances should always be kept away from light-coloured fabrics. As an alternative, spritz a hankie and tuck it into a pocket or into your bra - or (we do this sometimes) spray the underside of a collar, being careful not to get the 'juice' onto the visible part of the fabric.

EVERYTHING you ever *wanted* to know about FRAGRANCE

...But didn't know who to ask. These are the questions most often posed to us at The Perfume Society – with answers which we hope will tell you what you want to know about choosing, storing and wearing fragrance. (And if you've a question of your own? Email us at info@perfumesociety.org)

Q I love my friend's perfume. Why doesn't it smell as good on me?

A Everyone's body chemistry is different, influenced by hormones, skin type, what you eat, medications you may take and more. Simply adding a new vitamin or supplement to your well-being regime (if you have one!) can change how a fragrance smells on your skin. Even experts can't pinpoint which factors change perfume the most, or predict how a scent will be altered: it might become more sour, or more sweet. What is known is that deeper, richer notes – woods and ambery ingredients, for instance – won't change as much from person to person as do the fresher, more volatile ingredients such as citrus or lily. The bottom line is: don't ever buy a fragrance because you like it on a friend. More than that, never buy a fragrance without trying it on your own skin – full stop.

Q I hate my best friend's perfume and can hardly stand being in the same room as her. How can I make her give it up?

A We feel your pain – but we don't recommend a too-direct approach. Perfume is so inextricably linked with our sense of self that people can take criticism about their choice of scent very personally indeed. A kinder, gentler way is to collect a variety of samples of perfumes that you like (or can at least bear to be in the same room as!), whip them out next time you're having coffee and say something like: 'I've got all these samples – will you help me try them out…?' Make a mental note of which ones she likes the best and buy her a bottle. You can then say, 'That perfume smelled so amazing on you, I just had to get it' – while keeping the fingers of the other hand firmly crossed behind your back.

> *Never buy a fragrance because you like it on a friend*

Q I found an old bottle of perfume. Is it OK to use?

A Well, it won't kill you. But a lot depends on how well the fragrance was stored. If the scent's less than two years old, it's probably fine (especially if unopened). Test the scent on a tissue. If it seems to smell sour, or 'off', heat and oxidation may have broken down the fragrance molecules. The very best place to store fragrance to make it last is in a cool, dark place.

Q What can I do when I've applied too much perfume?

A One answer is to grab a lemon: the juice's acidity (more powerful than other citrus fruit) helps to cut the fragrance's oil. Wash with soap and water, then take off what's left with a cotton pad soaked in lemon juice.

Q Why does a perfume smell great on me at first but 'icky' later?

A Many perfumes are blended with notes – such as citrus – which give an initial zing. These evaporate quickly, though, allowing the middle and base notes to become more dominant: they're heavier and hang around longer. You've got to be sure you like all stages of a fragrance's 'journey' before buying it.

Q Can I wear more than one fragrance at a time?

A We believe this is going to be a massive trend. In the Middle East, women (and men) wear as many as seven different fragrances at a time, to create an entirely 'unique' and personal fragrance. This is pretty much heresy as far as the creators of perfumes are concerned – but certainly, in a region where people's clothing is very standardised – black gowns for women, white or beige for men – it's an effective form of self-expression. Jo Malone London™ is probably the only fragrance house that actively encourages 'fragrance combining', but we think its popularity is going to spread. What we do find works best, ourselves, is to combine two fragrances from within a family: pair a couple of Orientals, or a duo of fresh scents. It's fun, if you don't like the results you can wash them off (see page 167) – and you might come up with a combo that you love, love, love. But go lightly: you want a dab of this and a dab of that, rather than twice or three times the usual 'dose' you apply, if you don't want to overpower.

Q My tastes in fragrance change. Why?

A Most of us are fairly faithful to a particular family of fragrances – which is why when you understand the 'family' or 'families' you are consistently drawn to, it makes it easier to narrow down potential scent purchases. When shopping, start with scents in the same family as an old favourite. Seasonal allergies can make you smell things differently, though, as can a viral infection. (If that happens, don't instantly toss away your perfume: this should pass, once the allergies are under control or you're no longer sick.)

Rises in oestrogen during pregnancy also make you hypersensitive to odours: many women go right off their favourites at this time – although most find they can happily return to them after the baby's born. At menopause, the sense of smell can start to 'dim' slightly (although we believe it's possible to 'exercise' your sense of smell to ensure it maintains its sensitivity). At the same time, hormonal changes may also alter both your taste in fragrance and how it smells on the body: part of this is down to the fact that skin becomes drier and so fragrance doesn't 'cling' so well. (This is easily remedied: use a richer, unfragranced body moisturiser.)

As our lives evolve though, it's not uncommon for fragrance tastes to become more 'sophisticated'. Fruity-florals are 'younger', but those young women are rarely drawn to OTT Orientals, or sophisticated chypres. Just as we may become more discerning about wines, so it is with scent.

> *We believe it's possible to 'exercise' your sense of smell to ensure it maintains its sensitivity*

Q What's the difference between a perfume oil and an essential oil?

A Perfume oils are fragrance blends, in an oil base rather than an alcohol base, which can be applied directly to the skin. Please don't confuse these with essential oils: very few of those (with the exception of lavender and tea tree) can be applied neat to skin. Essential oils are the fragrant liquids extracted from the leaves, flowers, bark, seeds, buds, resins and stems of plants and need to be diluted – with alcohol (in a perfume) or base oil (such as sweet almond or jojoba) – before applying to the skin.

Q How can I make my fragrance last longer?

Layering with a perfume's matching lotion certainly works: we find when we do this that our chosen scent is sort of 'time-released' during the day, as the body warms up and cools down. But master perfumer Harry Fremont, based at Firmenich in New York, recommends applying an unscented, oil-based moisturiser before spritzing. Alternatively, trade up to a higher concentration of your chosen perfume (see pages 20–25 for more on this): the percentage of fragrance oil to alcohol base is higher, so the scent stays put for longer. Even the longest-lasting fragrance, though, probably won't be perceptible after more than about four hours without really sniffing your skin. If you don't want to lug around a bottle or a spray, we recommend the brilliant Travalo: a leak-proof mini-pump atomiser into which you can easily decant your favourite scent. Travalos now come in a wide range of colours (including black, gold and silver): we each have several, for our various different much-loved scents, in order to spritz on-the-go.

www.travalo.com

> *Even the longest-lasting fragrance probably won't be perceptible after more than about four hours*

Q When I'm perfume shopping, my nose gets 'tired'. What can I do to refresh it?

A Perfume stores and some counters supply coffee beans to 'refresh' the nose but to be honest, nice as coffee is to smell, we're not sure they're as effective as they're rumoured to be: coffee is just another strong scent to confuse your nose. It's better, we've found, to sniff your own skin (somewhere you haven't applied perfume) – the crook of the elbow is perfect – as it's a neutral, familiar scent. Be aware, though, that almost everyone's nose gets tired after smelling four or five different scents. Go easy and always take your time.

Q Should I buy perfume at Duty Free?

A If it's something you wear and love, yes, absolutely: you can save a little money or sometimes find exclusive editions. But something new…? We really recommend not: you can be halfway to Rio/Moscow/New York before the base notes really emerge – and that's the phase of the fragrance you'll live with the most. If you don't like that stage, there's no taking it back. But if you really, really, really have to make a snap decision, try the eau de toilette rather than the eau de parfum, as it will dry and develop faster, so you can make up your mind more swiftly.

Q What sort of perfumes should I wear for a job interview?

A When you feel 'comfortable' in an interview, you'll do your best, which means not only choosing the right clothing to make a good impression, but selecting your scent carefully. Is it OK to wear a fragrance to an interview? Absolutely – but the rule of thumb is to make sure it's on the light side and to apply just a touch. If you have a scent that makes you feel calm and relaxed, wear a drop of that. Otherwise, a very, very light floral can work, or just splash on a Cologne when you're getting dressed: the citrus notes will make you feel focused and alert, but the chances are by the time you get to your appointment, they'll have completely dissipated, as Colognes have a short life on the skin. But remember, in this situation less is more – so if you're anxious about overdoing it, go scent-free.

Q How relevant is it that a perfume is 'masculine', 'feminine' or 'shared'?

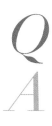

A Completely irrelevant, we say. A few centuries ago, there was no such thing as gender in perfume. It's true that not every man wants to waft around in a cloud of sugar violets and not that many women we know what to smell bracingly of a sea-breezy, ocean-inspired men's aftershave, but there is absolutely no reason why you shouldn't wear what you darned well like. We are very fond of (and wear) quite a few so-called 'men's fragrances' (Guerlain Vetiver, Dior Eau Sauvage) – and we have male friends who drench themselves in Guerlain Jicky for instance, and smell sublime, even though it's considered more of a feminine scent. An interesting development to come out of the more 'niche' end of perfumery is that many of these houses now use the phrase 'shared' to describe their perfumes and don't categorise them for men or women. They also decant their scents into bottles that could look equally good on either side of the bathroom shelf. And we're all for these barriers being broken down. Wear what you love. That's all that counts.

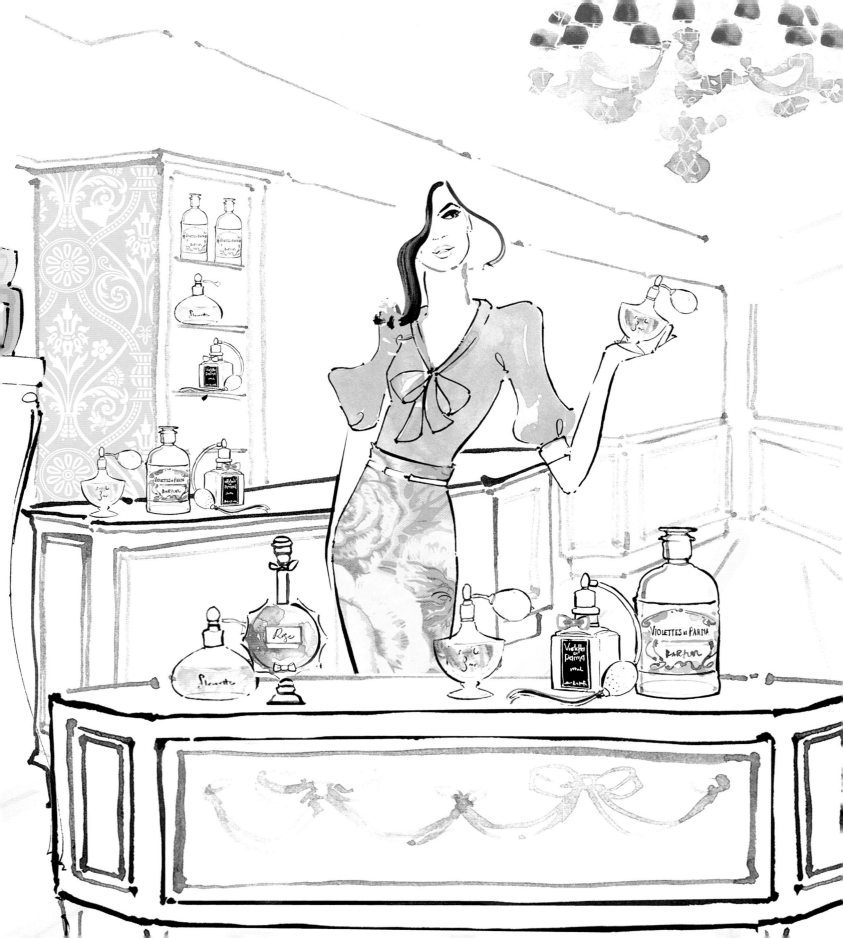

> *If you find a particular fragrance that seems to turn your partner on – we suggest you stockpile it…!*

Q Is perfume an aphrodisiac?

A Well, not strictly. There's no scientific evidence that fragrance does have an effect on sex drive, but we do know that fragrance can certainly make you feel sexier, and also works to 'get you in the mood' after a long and stressful day, perhaps simply by helping you to feel more relaxed. It's probably also got something to do with confidence: a lot of us feel more self-assured when we spray or dab on a particular fragrance. And if you do find a particular fragrance that seems to turn your partner on, we suggest you stockpile it…!

Q Why doesn't my favourite perfume smell like it used to?

A There are several reasons why this happens – and isn't it just so disappointing? Sometimes, companies do it for cost reasons – substituting a cheaper ingredient. It's generally assumed that's the case – but there are very often other factors at play. Sometimes, a once-plentiful natural ingredient becomes scarce, extinct even – or the authorities decide it's endangered and clamp down on its harvest. In terms of natural ingredients, there are differences from year to year, too, as well as from source to source: a crop of roses from one year may smell entirely different to the previous year's harvest. Vetiver from Haiti smells different to vetiver from India. And so on…

The other factor is that as more is understood about the potential for sensitivity or allergy to perfumes, increasingly tight restrictions are being placed on the quantity of that ingredient that is allowed to be used, by the International Fragrance Association (IFRA). Sometimes, there's an outright ban. At other times, the permitted level is reduced. Vanilla, oakmoss, jasmine, coumarin, styrax and opoponax are all either restricted, banned or under threat of restriction. It's a complete nightmare for 'noses' – who much of the time find themselves busily reformulating existing fragrances to bring them in line with the rules and regulations, when we're sure they'd much rather be pouring their creativity into new creations. The most talented perfumers in the haute parfumerie houses manage to rework their classics constantly, while keeping those treasures smelling just the same to us – adding in other ingredients to take the place of those that have been restricted. We take our hats off to them. But the bottom line is: if you think your favourite perfume doesn't smell like it used to, well, it probably doesn't. (And it may be time for something new…)

Q What are pheromones?

A Pheromones are biochemicals that signal our sexuality to others. Everyone has a unique pheromone signature: just ask any police dog! Pheromones are barely noticeable on a conscious level (you may occasionally get a whiff of 'muskiness' from an armpit or from someone's groin), but work on a primitive level. According to our friend Professor George Dodd (who actually produces fragrances based around pheromones, called Pheromol Factor), 'The sexually compatible enjoy each other's body odour, even without realising it. There's an odour conversation between them and that's what's meant by "sexual chemistry"'. Nowadays, that can be worked out scientifically. 'The output of pheromones starts with puberty, peaks in the late twenties, then diminishes,' explains George. He believes that it's possible to 'boost' natural pheromones by wearing a pheromone-mimicking fragrance. If you're interested, we suggest you try for yourself! (The niche perfumery brand Escentric Molecules, meanwhile – see page 119 – claim that their fragrances work with your own natural pheromones…)

Q Is there a difference between 'perfume' and 'fragrance'?

A Well, not really. You can use either word (though we find that women in the UK use the word 'perfume', while in the States 'fragrance' is more widely used). Strictly, though, 'perfume' is also a particular concentration: it's the most intense option (eau de parfum comes next, then eau de toilette – you can read more about how this works on page 21). 'Scent' is sometimes thought to be a bit of a downmarket word for describing fragrance/perfume – but we're not in the least snobby. If 'scent' is what you want to call it, great! We just want you to wear it and enjoy it as much as possible.

> *The sexually compatible enjoy each other's body odour, even without realising it*

Q I don't currently wear fragrance because I'm a bit shy of it. How should I start?

A We like this advice from perfumer Lyn Harris, of Miller Harris: 'If you've never worn fragrance, then approach it very simply as if it's an accessory that's going to "finish" your personality or your look and help you to feel good. To ease your way into a perfume, you could opt for a fresh citrus or a simple floral: these are always good bets'.

Q My favourite fragrance has been discontinued. Can I still find it?

A Welcome to Heartbreak Hotel. We hate it when this happens. There's always the possibility that you really will never find another bottle, but there's a lot you can do before that scenario has you reaching for your Kleenex. First of all, Google it. Don't just look at the shelves of your local department store and figure: that's it, over. Quite often, a fragrance that's been delisted by the major stores finds its way on to the internet via what's known as 'the grey market'. (The grey market refers to goods that are generally legitimately imported from abroad, carry a recognisable trademark or brand name and are sold at significant discounts outside of the manufacturer's normal channels of distribution.) Generally, we always recommend buying from department stores or well-known online retailers with links to actual stores: there are no guarantees of quality with the grey market. But desperate times call for desperate measures and if there's really no other way to find your discontinued perfume, it's worth a shot.

Also make it a No. 1 priority when you visit somewhere new to check out the perfume stores, chemists, beauty stores, department stores and anywhere else that has even the slimmest chance of carrying your favourite. And get in touch with the manufacturer: they can tell you if it's still being manufactured in your country and, if so, where it can be obtained. (Often a fragrance discontinued in one country is widely available elsewhere.) Check out eBay and other auction sites online. Rare gems often turn up but, again, there are no guarantees of quality here; if the bottle's been knocking around for a while, the contents may have changed quite a bit in character. And be aware that if it's highly sought-after, you may be up against fellow keen bidders, and end up having to pay through the nose (sorry).

Last but not least, there are some websites that carry rare fragrances: Direct Cosmetics (UK and USA), The Fragrance Factory (US), Enchanté (Canada). The downside is that even if you find the fragrance abroad, shipping restrictions on hazardous materials mean that it can nowadays be hard to get it mailed to you. And if you've no joy? FR.eD on The Perfume Society website (www.perfumesociety. org), our 'virtual' fragrance advisor, will make suggestions for your next love.

> *Oestrogen makes women more sensitive to smells*

Q Is it true that women have a keener sense of smell than men?

A According to Richard L. Doty, Director of the Smell and Taste Center at the University of Pennsylvania, USA, the answer is 'Yes'. Nobody's entirely sure why, though: it may be that women are simply encouraged to use the sense of smell more than men, through learning to cook, buying flowers, etc (not to mention becoming interested in the whole world of fragrance…). There are certainly hormonal fluctuations: oestrogen makes women more sensitive to smells in the first half of the menstrual cycle (and even more so in the early months of pregnancy – which is why so many women go right off their usual perfume then). Progesterone, meanwhile, decreases the ability to smell in the second half of the cycle.

Q Can I wear my perfume in the sun?

A Nononononoooooo! Really, please don't. With the exception of fragrances that advertise that they're 'safe' for sun exposure (some of the leading beauty brands occasionally bring these out), there are good reasons not to wear your perfume in the sun. Certain widely used fragrance ingredients – generally citrus-derived – contain psoralens, components that over-stimulate the pigment-producing cells, producing localised brown patches (which have the official medical name Berloque dermatitis), a streak of brown pigment akin to a raindrop running down a window pane. The solution? If you want to enjoy a summer fragrance in the sun, try spritzing it on your clothing rather than your skin. (Check first, of course, that it doesn't discolour the fabric: you can try it on a tissue.) Wear a ribbon around a wrist or your neck that has been drenched in scent à la Marie Antoinette and her mob. Drench some cotton wool in fragrance and tuck it into your bra (or your swimsuit, if you're not planning to get wet). And, of course, enjoy liberally after dark. Just be certain to cleanse away the fragrance next morning with a wet flannel before you go anywhere near the sun.

> *If you want to enjoy a summer fragrance in the sun, try spritzing it on your clothing rather than your skin*

Q Is the fragrance in a department store tester the same one I'm buying?

A Yes, absolutely. The whole idea is to give you a sense of what the fragrance smells like – and we can assure you that fragrance houses don't have special bottles for in-store spritzing. The only difference might be that the in-store tester, if it's been around for a while, may have been slightly affected by the light environment and even heat, both of which can damage a perfume. A clue can be if there's just a little of the perfume left in the bottle; you can always ask for a fresh tester to be put out (and any fragrance sales consultant really ought to oblige).

Q I'm very concerned about animal testing and cruelty. Do perfumes contain animal ingredients?

A Almost certainly not, nowadays. Although animal ingredients used to be among some of the most prized ingredients to perfumers – musk from musk deer, civet from the civet cat, castoreum from a sexual gland of the beaver – these have almost all been replaced by synthetic versions, which are a) cheaper, b) more reliable, and c) don't upset conservationists and those who (like us, and like you) are concerned about animal welfare. The one animal ingredient which is probably OK (unless you're a vegan) is ambergris: this is basically an ingredient regurgitated by sperm whales after eating cuttlefish. It's so rare and precious that, again, it's mostly synthetic recreations of ambergris that are used in modern perfumery. Because ingredients are so hush-hush, though, you can't be 100 per cent sure that a fragrance is free from animal ingredients – and even the customer careline probably can't tell you. We can only echo the advice of perfume expert Luca Turin: 'If you're really concerned about the possibility that something might have an animal ingredient, buy something recent and cheap'.

Q Is there any difference between a splash and a spray?

A There really shouldn't be, if they're the same concentration (ie if they're both eau de parfum, eau de toilette and so on). The difference is only in the application. But a spray bottle – because it's sealed all the time – may have a slightly longer shelf life, compared to an open-necked bottle in which the contents are exposed to fresh air each time you unstopper the lid. It's up to you whether you choose a spray or a splash – but if you go for the latter, always dab the stopper onto your body and wipe it on a tissue or handkerchief before re-stoppering, otherwise your body's natural oils can get into the perfume and may affect it, over time.

Q **Why are some ingredients listed on packaging and not others?**

A You've noticed that, unlike most beauty products, there's a relatively short list of what's in a fragrance (usually printed on the box but not the bottle itself). The perfume world has managed to side-step requirements for full labelling, which makers of products such as skin creams, shampoos and make-up have to abide by, because of the massive commercial sensitivity: for example, if Chanel had to list every ingredient in No. 5 on their packaging, their entire business would likely as not be destroyed by copyists faster than you can say 'Rue Cambon'. But by law, brands have to list some ingredients that are known sensitisers for some people; these ingredients include citral, limonene, isoeugenol, linalool, coumarin, benzyl alcohol, benzyl cinnamate and more. (You can Google a full rundown: just type in 'list of perfume allergens'.) Allergies and sensitivities, however, do affect only a tiny portion of the population, so ingredients are nothing to be paranoid about – although as we say earlier, do keep perfumed skin safely out of the sun.

> *If Chanel had to list every ingredient in No. 5 on their packaging, their entire business would be destroyed by copyists faster than you can say 'Rue Cambon'*

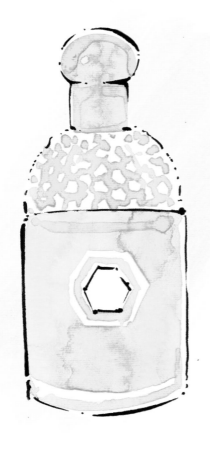

> " A woman's perfume tells more about her than her handwriting "

Christian Dior

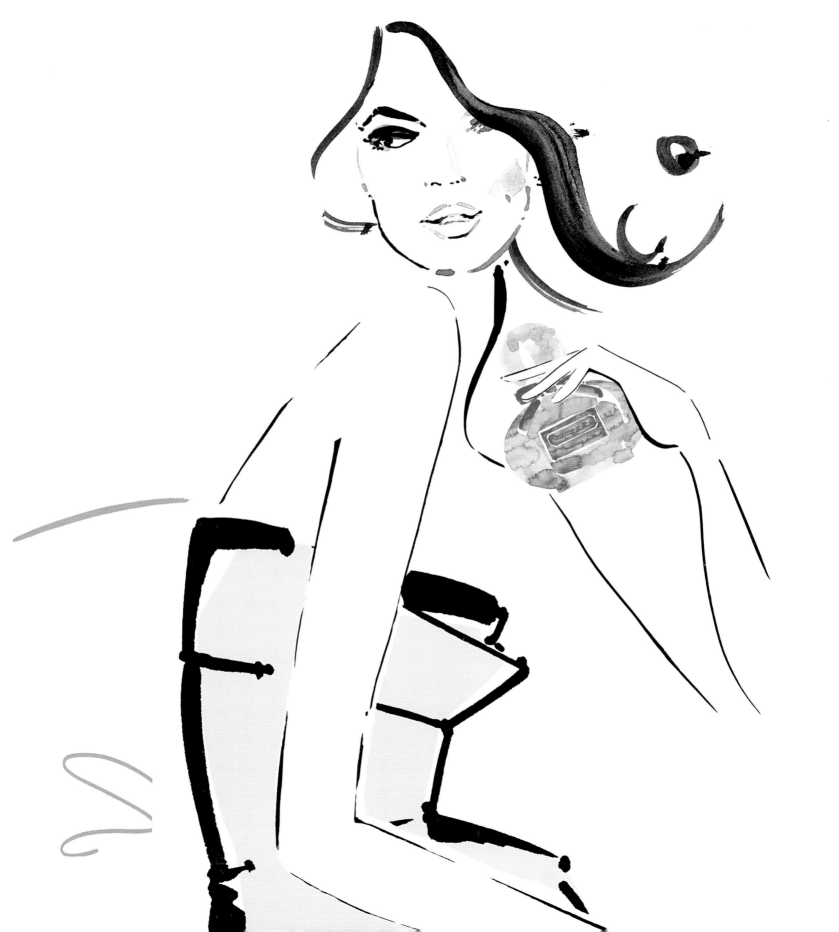

directory

4160 Tuesdays
www.4160tuesdays.com

Acqua di Parma
www.acquadiparma.com

AERIN
www.aerin.com

Agent Provocateur
www.agentprovocateur.com

Anastasia Brozler
www.scentlondon.co.uk

Annick Goutal
www.annickgoutal.com

Antonia's Flowers
www.antoniasflowers.com

Armani
www.armani.com

Atelier Cologne
www.ateliercologne.com

Aveda
www.aveda.co.uk
www.aveda.com

Balmain
www.balmain.com

Bobbi Brown
www.bobbibrown.co.uk
www.bobbibrown.com

The Body Shop
www.thebodyshop.co.uk
www.thebodyshop.com

Bois de Jasmin
www.boisdejasmin.com

Bottega Veneta
www.bottegaveneta.com

Boucheron
www.boucheron.com

Burberry
www.burberry.com

By Kilian
www.bykilian.com

By Terry
www.byterrydegunzburg.fr

Byredo
www.byredo.com

Cacharel
www.cacharel.com

Cafleurebon
www.cafleurebon.com

Calvin Klein
www.calvinklein.com

Candy Perfume Boy
www.thecandyperfumeboy.com

Caron
www.parfumscaron.com

Carthusia
www.carthusia.it

Cartier
www.cartier.co.uk
www.cartier.com

Carven
www.carven-parfums.com

Cerruti
www.cerruti1881fragrances.com

Chandler Burr
www.chandlerburr.com

Chanel
www.chanel.co.uk
www.chanel.com

Chloé
www.chloe.com

Clinique
www.clinique.co.uk
www.clinique.com

Clive Christian
www.clive.com

Comme des Garçons
www.comme-des-garcons-parfum.com

Courrèges
www.courreges.com

Creed
www.creedfragrances.co.uk
www.creedboutique.com

Davidoff
www.zinodavidoff.com

Dior
www.dior.com

Direct Cosmetics (UK/USA)
www.directcosmetics.com

DKNY
www.dkny.com

Dolce & Gabbana
www.dolcegabbana.com

The Dubai Perfume Souk
Sikkat al Khail Street, Deira (just east of the Gold Souk)

Editions de Parfums
Frederic Malle
www.fredericmalle.com

Elie Saab
www.eliesaab.com

Enchanté
www.eperfumes.ca

Escentric Molecules
www.escentric.com

Estee Lauder
www.esteelauder.co.uk
www.esteelauder.com

Etat Libre d'Orange
www.etatlibredorange.com

Farmaceutica di Santa Maria
Novella
www.smnovella.it

Firmenich
www.firmenich.com

Floris
www.florislondon.com

The Fragrance Factory
www.thefragrancefactory.com

Giorgio Beverly Hills
www.giorgiobeverlyhills.com

Givaudan
www.givaudan.com

Givenchy
www.givenchy.com

Grain de Musc
www.graindemusc.blogspot.co.uk

Grossmith
www.grossmithlondon.com

Guerlain
www.guerlain.com

Guy Larouche
www.guylaroche.com

Heeley Perfumes
www.jamesheeley.com

Hermès
www.hermes.com

Houbigant
www.houbigant-parfum.com

Houzz
www.houzz.com

Illuminum
www.illuminumfragrance.com

Institut Supérieur International du Parfum, de la Cosmétique et de l'Aromatique Alimentaire (ISIPCA)
www.isipca.fr

International Flavors and Fragrances (IFF)
www.iff.com

International Fragrance Association (IFRA)
www.ifraorg.org

International Perfume Bottle Association
www.perfumebottles.org

Issey Miyake
www.isseymiyake.com

Jardins d'Ecrivains
www.jardinsdecrivains.com

Jean Charles Brosseau
www.jcbrosseau.com

Jean Patou
www.jeanpatou.com

Jean Paul Gaultier
www.jeanpaulgaultier.com

Jennifer Lopez
www.jenniferlopezbeauty.com

Jimmy Choo
www.jimmychoo.com

Jo Malone London™
www.jomalone.co.uk
www.jomalone.com

Joop
www.coty.com/brands/joop

Jovoy
www.jovoyparis.com

Juliette Has A Gun
www.juliettehasagun.com

Katie Puckrik Smells
www.katiepuckriksmells.com

Kenzo
www.kenzoparfums.com

La Perla
www.laperla.com

Lalique
www.lalique.com

Lancôme
www.lancome.co.uk
www.lancome.com

Lanvin
www.lanvin.com

L'Artisan Parfumeur
www.artisanparfumeur.com

Le Labo
www.lelabofragrances.com

Les Senteurs
www.lessenteurs.com

Liz Earle
www.lizearle.com

L'O Profumo
www.loprofumo.com

L'Occitane
www.uk.loccitane.com
www.loccitane.com

Lolita Lempicka
www.parfumslolitalempicka.com

Londoner
www.bexlondon.com

Lorenzo Villoresi
www.lorenzovilloresi.it

Louis Vuitton
www.louisvuitton.com

Maison Francis Kurkdjian
www.franciskurkdjian.com

Maison Martin Margiela
www.maisonmartinmargiela-parfums.com

Mandy Aftel
www.aftelier.com

Marc Jacobs
www.marcjacobs.com

Marie-Antoinette
www.marieantoinetteparis.fr

Marni
www.marni.com

Mary Greenwell
www.marygreenwell.com

Mäurer & Wirtz 4711
www.4711.com

Memo Paris
www.memofragrances.com

Michael Kors
www.michaelkors.com

Miller Harris
www.millerharris.com

MiN NY
www.min.com

Molinard
www.molinard.com

Molton Brown
www.moltonbrown.co.uk
www.moltonbrown.com

Moschino
www.moschino.com

Narciso Rodriguez
www.narcisorodriguez.com

Natural Perfumers Guild
www.naturalperfumers.com

Nina Ricci
www.ninaricci.com

The Non-Blonde
www.thenonblonde.com

Nose
www.nose.fr

Now Smell This
www.nstperfume.com

The Organic Pharmacy
www.theorganicpharmacy.com

Ormonde Jayne
www.ormondejayne.com

Oscar de la Renta
www.oscardelarenta.com

Osswald (NYC)
www.osswaldnyc.com

Paco Rabane
www.pacorabanne.com

Penhaligon's
www.penhaligons.com

Perfume Posse
www.perfumeposse.com

Perfume Shrine
www.perfumeshrine.blogspot.
co.uk

Perfume Society
www.perfumesociety.org

Persolaise
www.persolaise.blogspot.co.uk

Pierre Dinand
www.pierre-dinand.com

Prada
www.prada.com

Reiss
www.reiss.com

Revlon
www.revlon.co.uk
www.revlon.com

Roads
www.roads.co/fragrance/

Robert Piguet
www.robertpiguetparfums.com

Robertet
www.robertet.com

Rochas
www.rochas.com

Roja Dove
www.rojadove.com

Roja Parfums
www.rojaparfums.com

Sarah Horowitz
www.sarahhorowitz.com

Scent Bar
www.luckyscent.com

The Scent Critic
www.thescentcritic.com

The Scented Salamander
www.mimifroufrou.com

Serge Lutens
www.sergelutens.com

Shay & Blue
www.shayandblue.com

Sisley
www.sisleyparis.com

Stella McCartney
www.stellamccartney.com

Strange Invisible Perfumes
www.siperfumes.com

Symrise
www.symrise.com

Takasago
www.takasago.com

Tauer Perfumes
www.tauerperfumes.com

Thierry Mugler
www.mugler.co.uk
www.mugler.com

Thirdman
www.thirdman.net

Tom Daxon
www.tomdaxon.com

Tom Ford
www.tomford.com

Travalo
www.travalo.com

Van Cleef & Arpels
www.vancleefarpels.com

Viktor & Rolf
www.viktor-rolf.com/en/
fragrance

Vintage Ad Browser
www.vintageadbrowser.com

Vintage in Print
www.vintageinprint.co.uk

Xerjoff
www.xerjoff.com

Yardley
www.yardleylondon.co.uk

Yohji Yamamoto
www.yohjiyamamotoparfums.
com

Yves Saint Laurent
www.yslbeauty.co.uk
www.yslbeauty.com

BOOKSHELF

Essence & Alchemy by Mandy Aftel

Glamour Icons: Perfume Bottle Design by Marc Rosen

Le Snob: Perfume by Dariush Alavi

Masters of Fashion Illustration by David Downton

Perfume: The Story of a Murderer by Patrick Süskind

The Perfume Lover: A Personal History of Scent by Denyse Beaulieu

Perfumes: The A-Z Guide by Luca Turin and Tania Sanchez

Remembering Smell: A Memoir of Losing – and Discovering – the Primal Sense by Bonnie Blodgett

The Scent Trail: A Journey of the Senses by Celia Lyttelton

Scents & Sensibilities: Creating Solid Perfumes for Well-Being by Mandy Aftel

index

A

absolutes 32, 65
accords 32
Acqua di Gioia (Armani) 103
Acqua di Parma: Colonia 10, 150
    Iris Nobile 100
advertising 76–79
Aftel, Mandy 70–71, 97
aftershave 22
age, and sense of smell 45
Agent Provocateur 102
aldehydes 32, 35, 49
Alien (Theirry Mugler) 143
ambergris 104
Ambre Gris (Balmain) 104
Anaïs Anaïs (Cacharel) 107
Angel (Thierry Mugler) 12, 34, 81, 140, 143, 145
animal testing 176
animalic notes 31, 32, 49
anosmia 32
Antonia's Flowers 103
Apps 29
Aqua Allegoria (Guerlain) 57, 60
Arabia 47, 48, 62
Armani: Acqua di Gioia 103
    Privé 6
aromatic 32
Aromatics Elixir (Clinique) 113
Arpège (Lanvin) 132
Atelier Cologne 85, 89
    Orange Sanguine 103
Aveda 96

B

Baccarat 49, 50, 82
Bacchanalia 47
Balmain 76
    Ambre Gris 104
    Vent Vert 104
Balmain, Pierre 81
balsamic 33
base notes 29, 31, 33
Be Delicious (DKNY) 117
Beach (Bobbi Brown) 104
Beauharnais, Josephine de 49
Beaulieu, Denyse 31
Beaux, Ernest 49, 112, 113
Bendeth, Marian 37
benzoin 33, 35
bergamot 33, 53, 54, 59, 63, 71
bespoke fragrances 92–97
Beverley Hills (Giorgio) 123
Biguine, Anaïs 87
Birkin, Jane 94
Black Orchid (Tom Ford) 144
Blodgett, Bonnie 45
bloggers 162–165
blotters 28–29, 35, 40
Bluebell (Penhaligon's) 140
Bobby Brown, Beach 104
body heat and perfume 21
Body Shop, White Musk 105
Bois de Jasmin 40, 66
Bonbon (Viktor & Rolf) 80
Botanical Essence No. 15 (Liz Earle) 133
Bottega Veneta, Eau de Parfum 105
bottles 40, 49, 50, 80–83
Bouché, René 79
Boucheron, Boucheron 106
Bouquet, Carole 76
Bourjois 50
brands 65
Brosseau, Jean Charles, Ombre Rose L'Original 128
Brozler, Anastasia 96–97
Burberry 82
Burr, Chandler 57, 132
Burri, Edmond 58
Byredo, Flowerhead 106

C

Cacharel, Anaïs Anaïs 107
Caesar, Julius 47
Café Rose (Tom Ford) 144
Calandre (Paco Rabanne) 81
Calèche (Hermès) 127
Calvin Klein: ck one 51, 107
    Eternity 107
    Obsession 11, 51, 81, 108
Calyx (Clinique) 59, 114
camphorous 33
Candy (Prada) 140
Cardin, Pierre 81
Carnal Flower (Editions de Parfums Frederic Malle) 118
Carnegie, Hattie 82
Caron, Françoise 100, 128
Caron, Tabac Blond 108
Carthusia, Fiori di Capri 12
Cartier 57, 65
    Must de Cartier 109
    La Panthère 109
Carven 50
    Ma Griffe 110
    Le Parfum 110
castoreum 32
Catholicism 47
Cavallier, Jacques 57, 130
cedarwood 35
celebrity scents 8, 128
Cerruti, Cerruti 1881 13
Cervasel, Christophe 85
Chanel 54, 57, 65, 82
    advertising 76
    Chanel No. 5 21, 32, 49, 50, 72, 76, 112, 177
    Chanel No. 19 12, 35, 112, 115, 150
    Chanel No. 22 113
    Coco 11, 51, 110
    Coco Mademoiselle 112
    Cuir de Russie 34
    Les Exclusifs 6
    ingredients 63
    layering 23
    Pour Monsieur 150
    Sycomore 13
Chanel, Gabrielle 'Coco' 21, 49, 50, 73, 112
Chant, Bernard 103
Charlie Blue (Revlon) 141
China 46
Chloé, Chloé 11
Choo, Jimmy 130
Christian, Clive, No. 1 114
Chypre (François Coty) 12, 33
chypre fragrances 12, 13, 19, 33, 54
citrus notes 21
ck one (Calvin Klein) 51, 107
Classique (Jean Paul Gaultier) 130
Cleopatra 46, 47
Clinique: Aromatics Elixir 113
    Calyx 114
Clive Christian No. 1 114
clothing 26, 28, 165
CO_2 extraction 65
Coco (Chanel) 11, 51, 110
Coco Mademoiselle (Chanel) 112
cold pressing 65
La Collection Privée (Dior) 6
Colonia (Acqua di Parma) 150
composition of fragrance 31, 33
concretes 32, 65

conifer oils 33
Cool Water (Davidoff) 151
Coty, François 49, 50
  Chypre 12, 33
Courrèges, Empreinte 12
Creed, Love in White 114
Crete 46
Crusaders 48
Cuir de Russie (Chanel) 34
Cyprus 48

D

Daisy (Marc Jacobs) 80, 136
Dalí, Salvador 76
Daphne odora 72
Davidoff, Cool Water 151
Daxon, Tom 91
de la Renta, Oscar, Live in
  Love 10
decants 33
deodorant 26
Dinand, Pierre 80–81, 146
Dior 65, 76
  La Collection Privée 6
  Diorama 50
  Diorella 50, 76, 115
  Diorissimo 50, 76, 115
  Eau Sauvage 80, 81, 151,
    170
  J'Adore 116
  Miss Dior 12, 50, 76, 116
  Poison 51, 116
Dior, Christian 50, 81, 178
DKNY, Be Delicious 117
Dodd, Professor George 6,
  173
Dolce & Gabbana: Light Blue
117
  The One 11
Dot (Marc Jacobs) 80
Doty, Richard L. 175
Dove, Roja 29, 41, 82, 90, 96,
142
Downton, David 79
dry-down 33

the Dubai Perfume Souk 161
Dubreuil, Karine 57
duty free 50, 170
Dzing! (L'Artisan Parfumeur)
13

E

Earle, Liz, Botanical Essence
  No.15 133
eau d'abondance 22–23
eau de cologne 10, 22, 23,
  49, 54
Eau de Parfum (Bottega
  Veneta) 105
eau de parfum 21, 22, 23, 38
eau de toilette 10, 21, 22, 23
Eau d'Hadrien (Annick
  Goutal) 102
Eau du Soir (Sisley) 143
eau fraîche 22, 23
eau généreuse 22–23
Eau Sauvage (Dior) 80, 81,
  151, 170
Eau Universelle (L'Occitane)
  10
Editions de Parfums Frederic
  Malle: Carnal Flower 118
  Musc Ravageur 118
Edwards, Michael 125
Egypt, Ancient 46, 47, 62
Elie Saab Le Parfum 118
Elizabeth, Queen of Hungary
  48
Elizabeth Arden 82
Ellena, Jean-Claude 56, 57
Emporio Armani, Diamonds
  11
Empreinte (Courrèges) 12
Encre Noir (Lalique) 153
enfleurage 63, 65
English Lavender (Yardley)
  146
Equipage (Hermès) 153
Erté 79
Escentric Molecules,

Molecule 01 119
Essence (Narciso Rodriguez)
  138
essential oils 63, 65, 169
Estée Lauder 74, 76, 131
  Knowing 36, 119
  Oriental Youth Dew 50
  White Linen 120
  Youth Dew 120
Etat Libre d'Orange, Jasmine
  & Cigarette 120
Eternity (Calvin Klein) 107
eucalyptus 63, 71
evaluators 65–66
Les Exclusifs (Chanel) 6
expression 65
extrait de parfum 21

F

factice 33
families, fragrance 8–13, 168
Fargeon, Jean-Louis 48
Farmaceutica di Santa Maria
  Novella, Florence 161
Féminité du Bois (Serge
  Lutens) 142
Femme (Rocha) 36
Fidji (Guy Laroche) 126
Figue Amère (Miller Harris)
  138
Fiori di Capri (Carthusia) 12
Firenze (Lorenzo Villoresi) 135
Firmenich 35, 55, 58, 65
First (Van Cleef & Arpels) 145
fixatives 31, 33
flanker 33
floral fragrances 10, 19
floralcy 33
floriental fragrances 10, 11, 19
Floris 96
Flower by Kenzo 131
Flowerbomb (Viktor & Rolf)
  145
Flowerhead (Byredo Parfums)
  106

Ford, Tom: Black Orchid 144
  Café Rose 144
  Grey Vetiver 154
  Tobacco Vanille 12
fougère fragrances 13, 33
Fougère Royale (Houbigant)
  13, 33, 49
4160 Tuesdays (Sarah
  McCartney) 85
4711 (Wilhelm Meulhens) 100
Fracas (Piguet) 74, 142
fragrance: construction 31
  families 8–13, 168
  fragrance houses 65–66
  fragrance wardrobes 36–41
Fragrance Foundation
  Awards 70, 82, 103
France 48, 54, 63
frangipani 35
frankincense 33, 71
FR.eD 29, 174
Fremont, Harry 169
French Revolution 48–49
fresh fragrances 10, 19
Frolova, Victoria 40, 164

G

Ganter, Sylvie 85
Gardenia 35, 73
Gaultier, Jean Paul, Classique
  130
Gentleman Only (Givenchy)
  153
gifts, fragrances as 35
Giorgio, Beverley Hills 51,
  123
Givaudan 29, 54, 55, 58, 65
Givenchy: Gentleman Only
  153
  Ysatis 51, 80
Glasser, Azzi 38
Glow (J. Lo) 128
Glowing (J. Lo) 80
Goswell, Rebecca 88
gourmand fragrances 12, 19,

34

Goutal, Annick, Eau
d'Hadrien 102

Goya 50

Grasse, France 48, 54, 63

Greece, Ancient 46

Greenwell, Mary 89
Plum 137

Greves, Jean-Christophe le
91

Grey Flower (Reiss) 140

Grey Vetiver (Tom Ford) 154

Grojsman, Sophia 59, 114,
120, 132, 146

Grossmith 86

Gruau, René 76

guerilla sprayers 6, 28

Guerlain 50, 54, 55, 57–60, 90,
96
Après L'Ondée 146
Aqua Allegoria 57, 60
Guerlain Shalimar 35
Guerlinade 32
Habit Rouge 58
Idylle 57
Iris Ganache 58
Jicky 49, 50, 60, 124, 170
L'Heure Bleu 60, 123
La Petite Robe Noire 57, 60
layering 23
Mitsouko 38, 50, 60, 124
Quand Vient la Pluie 58
Samsara 51, 125
Shalimar 11, 50, 57, 60, 125
Vetiver 170
Vol de Nuit 13, 50

Guerlain, Aimé 49, 59

Guerlain, Jacques 58, 59, 124,
125

Guerlain, Jean-Paul 57, 58,
125

Gunzburg, Terry de 106

H

Habit Rouge (Guerlain) 58

hair 97

Hall, Jerry 50

Hammam Bouquet
(Penhaligon's) 11

Harris, Lyn 94–95, 138, 173

Heeley Perfumes 87

Henin, François 88

Hennessy, Kilian 85

herbal fragrances 34

Hermès 56, 57, 65, 79
Calèche 127
Equipage 153
24 Faubourg 126

hexane 32, 63

history of perfume 46–51

Homme (Yohji) 154

Horowitz, Sarah 97

Houbigant, Fougère Royale
13, 33, 49

Hugo, Victor 156

Hungary water 48

hyacinth 63

I

Idylle (Guerlain) 57

Illuminum 87, 96
White Gardenia Petals 10,
127

incense 46, 47–48, 62

independent perfumeries
84–91

indolic 34

ingredients 21, 52–55, 172, 177

International Flavors &
Fragrances (IFF) 55, 65, 91

International Fragrance
Association (IFRA) 21, 172

International Perfume Bottle
Association 82

Iris Ganache (Guerlain) 58

Iris Nobile (Acqua di Parma)
100

Italy 48

J

Jacobs, Marc: Daisy 80, 136
Dot 80

J'Adore (Dior) 116

Jardins d'Ecrivains 87

jasmine 10, 53, 54

Jasmine & Cigarette (Etat
Libre d'Orange) 120

jewellery, and perfume 45

Jicky (Guerlain) 49, 50, 60,
124, 170

Jimmy Choo, Jimmy Choo
130

Jo Malone London™ 131, 168

Joop, Joop! Homme 13

Jovoy, Paris 88, 160

Joy (Jean Patou) 128

Juliette Has A Gun 88

Juniper Sling (Penhaligon's)
154

K

Karl Lagerfeld 82

Keller, Helen 6, 25, 42

Kenzo, Flower by Kenzo 131

By Kilian 85

Knowing (Estée Lauder) 36,
119

Kors, Michael, Very
Hollywood 10

Kurkdjian, Francis 33, 57, 66,
88
Oud 135
perfumes by 89, 110, 123,
134

L

La Panthère (Cartier) 109

La Perla, La Perla 132

La Petite Robe Noire
(Guerlain) 57, 60

L'Air de Rien (Miller Harris) 94

L'Air du Temps (Nina Ricci)
126, 139

L'Artisan Parfumeur: Dzing!
13
Mure et Muse 133

L'Eau d'Issey (Issey Miyake)
51, 127

L'Étrange Fleur (Paul Poiret)
49

L'Heure Bleu (Guerlain) 60,
123

L'O Profumo, Florence 161

L'Occitane 23, 57, 65
La Collection de Grasse
Magnolia & Mûre 134
Eau Universelle 10

La Perla (La Perla) 132

Lady Million (Paco Rabanne)
11, 139

Lalique 49, 50, 139
Encre Noir 153

Lalique, Marc 82

Lalique, René 82

Lancôme: Magie Noire 80
Ô de Lancôme 10
Trésor 132

language of scent 30–35

Lanvin 50, 76
Arpège 132

Laroche, Guy, Fidji 126

Lathyrus odoratus 73

Lauder, Aerin 38

Lauder, Estée 38, 50, 120
see also Estée Lauder

Lauder, Evelyn 74

Laurent, Mathilde 57, 109

lavandin 33

lavender 33, 35, 38, 53, 54

layering 23, 169

leathery 34

Lempicka, Lolita, Lolita
Lempicka 12, 134

Light Blue (Dolce &
Gabbana) 117

lilac 34, 35

lily of the valley 35, 62–63

limbic system 44

Lime, Basil & Mandarin (Jo

Malone London™) 131
linden blossom 63
linear perfumes 34
Lyttelton, Celia 55
Live in Love (Oscar de la Renta) 10
Lolita Lempicka (Lolita Lempicka) 12, 134
Londoner 88
Lopez, Jennifer: Glow 128
    Glowing 80
Louis Vuitton 57, 65
Louis XIV 48
Love in White (Creed) 114
Lutens, Serge, Féminité du Bois 142

M

Ma Griffe (Carven) 110
McCartney, Sarah 85
McKnight, Sam 72–75
Madonna 74
Magie Noire (Lancôme) 80
Maitres-Gantiers 48
Malle, Frederic 6, 81
    Carnal Flower 123
    Editions de Parfums 51, 86
    Musc Ravageur 118
Malone, Jo 168
    Lime, Basil & Mandarin 131
Margiela, Martin 136
Marie Antoinette 33, 48, 49
Marie-Antoinette, Paris 160
Mark Antony 46, 47
marketing 50, 51
Marni, Marni 137
Master Perfumer 35
Medici, Queen Catherine de 48
MEMO Paris (John & Clara Molloy) 89
memories and smells 42–45
men's fragrances 13, 148–55, 170

Mesopotamians 46
Meulhens, Wilhelm, 4711 100
Middle Ages 47
Miller Harris 173
    Figue Amère 138
    L'Air de Rien 94
mimosa 63
MiN NY, New York 159
Miss Dior (Dior) 12, 50, 76, 116
Mitsouko (Guerlain) 38, 50, 60, 124
Miyake, Issey, L'Eau d'Issey 51, 127
Molecule 01 (Escentric Molecules) 119
Molloy, John and Clara 89
Molton Brown, Rogart 13
Momo, Sergio 91
Moschino, Cheap & Chic 10
Mugler, Thierry: Alien 143
    Angel 12, 34, 81, 140, 143, 145
Mure et Muse (L'Artisan Parfumeur) 133
Musc Ravageur (Editions de Parfums Frederic Malle) 118
Museum of Arts and Design, New York 57, 132
musk 32, 33, 35, 49
Must de Cartier (Cartier) 109

N

Nagel, Christine 57
Napoleon 49
narcissus 63, 73
nasal sprays 45
Natural Perfumers Guild 70
natural perfumery 70–71
Nero, Emperor 47
neroli 34, 53, 54, 71
The Non-Blonde 41
noses 34, 45, 54, 56–61, 65–66

notes 31, 32, 168
Nuit de Chine (Paul Poiret) 49
No.1 (Clive Christian) 114

O

Ô de Lancôme (Lancôme) 10
oakmoss 33, 60
Obsession (Calvin Klein) 11, 51, 81, 108
olfactory receptors 44, 45
Ombre Mercure (By Terry) 106
Ombre Rose L'Original (Jean Charles Brosseau) 128
The One (Dolce & Gabbana) 11
Opium (YSL) 50, 80
orange blossom 34, 35
orange flower water 63
orange flowers 59
Orange Sanguine (Atelier Cologne) 103
Organic Glam Citron (The Organic Pharmacy) 10
Organic Pharmacy (The), Organic Glam Citron 10
oriental fragrances 11, 19, 33, 35, 41, 55
Oriental Youth Dew (Estée Lauder) 50
Ormonde Jayne 90, 96
orris root 33
Osswald, New York 159
Oud (Maison Francis Kurkdjian) 135
ozonic 35

P

Paco Rabanne: Calandre 81
    Lady Million 11, 139
parfum 21, 22, 38
Le Parfum (Carven) 110
Le Parfum (Elie Saab) 118

Paris (YSL) 146
Parquet, Paul 49
patchouli 33, 35, 71
Patou, Jean 50, 65
    Joy 82, 128
Pelargonium 'Attar of Roses' 73
Penhaligon's: Bluebell 140
    Hammam Bouquet 11
    Juniper Sling 154
perfume (parfum) 21, 22, 38
perfume oils 169
perfume pyramid 31
The Perfume Society 28, 29, 45, 165
perfumers 56–61, 65–66, 81
Perfumery School, Switzerland 58
petitgrain 53, 54
pheromones 173
Piguet, Fracas 74, 142
Pilkington, Linda 90, 96
pine 33
Plum (Mary Greenwell) 137
Poiret, Paul 49, 50
    L'Ètrange Fleur 49
    Nuit de Chine 49
Poison (Dior) 51, 116
Polge, Jacques 57, 61
Polyanthus tuberosa 74
pomanders 47
portraits, perfume 14–19
Pour Monsieur (Chanel) 150
powdery 35
power perfumes 51
Prada: Candy 12, 140
    Pour Homme 13
preferences, smell 44
Privé (Armani) 6
Provenzano, Christian 102
psychology of scent 42–45
pulse points 21, 41

Q

Quand Vient la Pluie

Q

Quand Vient la Pluie (Guerlain) 58

R

rare fragrances 174
Reiss, Grey Flower 140
religious ceremonies 47–48
Renaissance 48
Revlon, Charlie Blue 141
Ricci, Nina 82, 88
  L'Air du Temps 126, 139
Ricci, Romano 88
rich fragrances 35
Risqué (Roja Parfums) 142
Rive Gauche (YSL) 80, 146
Roads, White Noise 141
Robert, François 88, 89
Robert, Guy 81, 127, 153
Robertet 65
Rochas, Femme 36
Rochas, Helene 81
Rochas, Marcel 81
Rodriguez, Narciso, Essence 138
Rogart (Molton Brown) 13
Roja Parfums 29, 41, 82, 90
  Risqué 142
Roman Catholics 47
Romans 47
room-rockers 51
rose water 48, 63
Rosen, Marc 82
roses 10, 53, 54, 74
rosewood 35
Roudnitska, Edmond 81, 115, 151

S

Saab, Elie, Le Parfum 118
Saks Fifth Avenue 82

Salisbury, Lauren 66
Samsara (Guerlain) 51, 125
sandalwood 35, 53, 55, 63
Sarcococca hookeriana var. humilis 74
Scent Bar, Los Angeles 160
Schiaparelli, Elsa 50, 76
seasons 38
seductive scents 41, 172
Les Senteurs, London 158
Shalimar (Guerlain) 11, 50, 57, 60, 125
Shay & Blue, Suffolk Lavender 13
Sheldrake, Christopher 57
shopping for perfume 26–29, 38, 40–41, 71, 169, 176
shops, perfume 158–161
signature scents 36–41, 92–97
sillage 35
Sisley, Eau du Soir 143
skin types and fragrances 21, 23, 167
smell, sense of 6, 45, 175
smoking 44
soapy fragrances 35
The Social Issues Research Centre 44
soliflore 35
Solon 46–47
solvent extraction 63, 65
spices 35
spill 35
steam distillation 63, 65
Stephanotis floribunda 74
storing fragrance 167
Strange Invisible Perfumes, Los Angeles 159
strength of perfumes 20–23
Süe, Louis 82
Suffolk Lavender (Shay & Blue) 13
supercritical fluid extraction 65
Süskind, Patrick, Perfume 56

Sycomore (Chanel) 13
Symons, Arthur (William) 69
Symrise 65
synthetic notes 32

T

Tabac Blond (Caron) 108
Takasago 65
Tallien, Madame 48
taste 45
Tauer Perfumes 90
terroir 54
By Terry, Ombre Mercure 106
Thirdman 91
tiaré 35, 52, 55, 71
Tobacco Vanille (Tom Ford) 12
tolu balsam 35
tonka 52, 55
Trachelospermum jasminoides 75
Tresor (Lancôme) 59, 132
tuberose 34, 35, 63
Turin, Dr Luca 19, 124, 134, 151, 176
24 Faubourg (Hermès) 126

U

Union Fragrance 96

V

Van Cleef & Arpels, First 145
vanilla 35, 53, 55
Venice 48
Vent Vert (Balmain) 104
Very Hollywood (Michael Kors) 10
vetiver 52, 55, 63
Vetiver (Guerlain) 170
Victorians 49

Viktor & Rolf: Bonbon 80
  Flowerbomb 145
Villoresi, Lorenzo 97
  Firenze Piper Negrum 135
virtual fragrance advisors 29
Vol de Nuit (Guerlain) 13, 50

W

Warhol, Andy 76
Wasser, Thierry 54, 57–60, 96, 124
weather 38, 41, 175
white floral scents 35, 55
White Gardenia Petals (Illuminum) 10, 127
White Linen (Estée Lauder) 120
White Musk (The Body Shop) 105
White Noise (Roads) 141
woody fragrances 13, 19, 35

X

Xerjoff 91

Y

Yardley 50
  English Lavender 146
ylang ylang 53, 55, 63
Yohji, Homme 154
Youth Dew (Estée Lauder) 120
Ysatis (Givenchy) 51, 80
YSL: Opium 50, 80
  Paris 146
  Rive Gauche 80, 146

Top 100 perfumes to try before you die

1. 4711 (Fresh)

2. Acqua di Parma Iris Nobile (Chypre)

3. Agent Provocateur (Chypre)

4. Annick Goutal Eau d'Hadrien (Fresh)

5. Antonia's Flowers (Floral)

6. Armani Acqua di Gioia (Fresh)

7. Atelier Cologne Orange Sanguine (Fresh)

8. Balmain Ambre Gris (Oriental)

9. Balmain Vent Vert (Floral)

10. Bobbi Brown Beach (Floral)

11. The Body Shop White Musk (Floriental)

12. Bottega Veneta Eau de Parfum (Chypre)

13. Boucheron Boucheron (Floral)

14. By Terry Ombre Mercure (Floral)

15. Byredo Flowerhead (Floral)

16. Cacharel Anaïs Anaïs (Floral)

17. Calvin Klein ck one (Fresh)

18. Calvin Klein Eternity (Floral)

19. Calvin Klein Obsession (Oriental)

20. Caron Tabac Blond (Chypre)

21. Cartier La Panthère (Chypre)

22. Cartier Must de Cartier (Oriental)

23. Carven Le Parfum (Floral)

24. Carven Ma Griffe (Chypre)

25. Chanel Coco (Oriental)

26. Chanel Coco Mademoiselle (Chypre)

27. Chanel No. 5 (Floral)

28. Chanel No. 19 (Floral)

29. Chanel No. 22 (Floral)

30. Clinique Aromatics Elixir (Chypre)

31. Clinique Calyx (Floral)

32. Clive Christian No. 1 (Floral)

33. Creed Love In White (Floral)

34. Dior Diorella (Fresh)

35. Dior Diorissimo (Floral)

36. Dior J'Adore (Floral)

37. Dior Miss Dior (Chypre)

38. Dior Poison (Floral)

39. DKNY Be Delicious (Floral)

40. Dolce & Gabbana Light Blue (Floral)

41. Editions de Parfums Frederic Malle Carnal Flower (Floral)

42. Editions de Perfums Frederic Malle Musc Ravageur (Oriental)

43. Elie Saab Le Parfum (Floral)

44. Escentric Molecules Molecule 01 (Woody)

45. Estée Lauder Knowing (Chypre)

46. Estée Lauder White Linen (Floral)

47. Estée Lauder Youth Dew (Oriental)

48. d'Orange Jasmine & Cigarette (Woody)

49. Giorgio Beverley Hills (Floral)

50. Guerlain L'Heure Bleu (Oriental)

51. Guerlain Jicky (Oriental)

52. Guerlain Mitsouko (Chypre)

53. Guerlain Samsara (Oriental)

54. Guerlain Shalimar (Oriental)

55. Guy Laroche Fidji (Floral)

56. Hermès 24 Faubourg (Chypre)

57. Hermès Calèche (Floral)

58. Illuminum White Gardenia Petals (Floral)

59. Issey Miyake L'Eau d'Issey (Fresh)

60. J.Lo Glow (Floral)

61. Jean Charles Brosseau Ombre Rose L'Original (Floral)

62. Jean Patou Joy (Floral)

63. Jean Paul Gaultier Classique (Floriental)

64. Jimmy Choo Jimmy Choo (Chypre)

65. Jo Malone London™ Lime, Basil & Mandarin (Fresh)

66. Kenzo Flower by Kenzo (Floral)

67. La Perla La Perla (Chypre)

68. Lancôme Trésor (Floral)

69. Lanvin Arpège (Floral)

70. L'Artisan Parfumeur Mûre et Musc (Floral)

71. Liz Earle Botanical Essence No. 15 (Oriental)

72. L'Occitane en Provence La Collection de Grasse Magnolia & Mûre (Oriental)

73. Lolita Lempicka Lolita Lempicka (Gourmand)

74. Lorenzo Villoresi Piper Nigrum (Oriental)

75. Maison Francis Kurkdjian Oud (Woody)

76. Maison Martin Margiela (Woody)

77. Marc Jacobs Daisy (Floral)

78. Marni Marni (Woody)

79. Mary Freenwell Plum (Chypre)

80. Miller Harris Figue Amère (Floral)

81. Narciso Rodriguez Essence (Floral)

82. Nina Ricci L'Air du Temps (Floral)

83. Paco Rabanne Lady Million (Floral)

84. Penhaligon's Bluebell (Floral)

85. Prada Candy (Gourmand)

86. Reiss Grey Flower (Oriental)

87. Revlon Charlie Blue (Floral)

88. Roads White Noise (Fresh)

89. Robert Piguet Fracas (Floral)

90. Roja Parfums Risqué (Chypre)

91. Serge Lutens Féminité du Bois (Woody)

92. Sisley Eau du Soir (Chypre)

93. Thierry Mugler Alien (Oriental)

94. Tom Ford Black Orchid (Oriental)

95. Tom Ford Café Rose (Floriental)

96. Van Cleef & Arpels First (Floral)

97. Viktor & Rolf Flowerbomb (Floral)

98. Yardley English Lavender (Fresh)

99. YSL Paris (Floral)

100. YSL Rive Gauche (Floral)

The Men's Room

1. Acqua di Parma Colonia (Fresh)

2. Chanel Pour Monsieur (Fougère)

3. Davidoff Cool Water (Fresh)

4. Dior Eau Sauvage (Fresh)

5. Givenchy Gentleman Only (Woody)

6. Hermès Equipage (Fougère)

7. Lalique Encre Noir (Woody)

8. Penhaligon's Juniper Sling (Woody)

9. Tom Ford Grey Vetiver (Woody)

10. Yohji Homme (Woody)

picture credits

p5: Ateli/istock

p6–7: Ateli/istock

p10, 11, 12, 13: Ateli/istock

p14 (clockwise from top): powdr_dayz/istock; A_teen/istock; kazoka30/istock

p15: nickpo/istock; robcocquyt/istock; Alexander Raths/Shutterstock; ac_bnphotos/istock; Aprilphoto/Shutterstock

p16: RG-vc/Shutterstock; pidjoe/istock; ONimages/istock; SerenDigital/istock; dtimiraos/istock

p17 (top to bottom): left column: Alan_Lagadu/istock; mariusz_prusaczyk/istock; naphtalina/istock; AndreaAstes/istock

right column: Kate Sinclair/FilmMagic; intrepidina/Shutterstock; Stan Honda/AFP/Getty Images; wavebreakmedia/Shutterstock; sf_foodphoto/istock

p18 (clockwise from top): fotograv/istock; xyzphoto/istock; Jpecha/istock; Andrey Bandurenko/Fotolia

p19 (top to bottom): PapaBear/istock; MKucova/istock; ryasick/istock; oscarhdez/istock; Vasiliki Varvaki/Getty Images

p26: Yonel/istock

p27: Michael Ochs Archives/Corbis

p28: kubais/Shutterstock

p30–31: Teri Caviston/Shutterstock

p39: Courtesy of AERIN, LLC

p41: RDPR Group Ltd

p46 (left to right): Lance Lee/Dreamstime; Marilyn Barbone/Dreamstime; Dea Picture Library/Getty Images; Ask me no more,

1906 (oil on canvas), Alma-Tadema, Sir Lawrence (1836-1912)/Private Collection/The Bridgeman Art Library; Shutterstock/mishabender; Ashwin Kharidehal Abhirama/Dreamstime

p47: Roses of Heliogabalus, 1888 (oil on canvas), Alma-Tadema, Sir Lawrence (1836-1912)/Private Collection/© Whitford Fine Art, London, UK/Bridgeman Images; Stock Montage/Getty Images; Photocuisine/Alamy; Sarah Marchant/Dreamstime; Ugurhan Betin/Getty Images; Paola Bona/Shutterstock

p48: Ivy Close Images/Alamy; BOTTLE BRUSH/Balan Madhavan/Alamy; Jon Arnold Images Ltd/Alamy; Jozef Sedmak/Alamy; Francesco Alessi/Dreamstime; Angela Conrady/Getty Images; Portrait of Louis XIV (1638-1715) (oil on canvas), Rigaud, Hyacinthe (1659-1743) /Prado, Madrid, Spain/Giraudon/Bridgeman Images

p49: Author's Image Ltd/Alamy; Dziewul/Dreamstime; Napoleon and Josephine Melodrama, c.1898 (colour litho), French School, (19th century)/ Private Collection/DaTo Images/Bridgeman Images; The Young Queen Victoria (1819-1901) (panel), Winterhalter, Franz Xaver (1806-73) (circle of)/ Private Collection/Photo © Philip Mould Ltd, London/Bridgeman Images; Peter Stone/Alamy; Apic/Getty Images; Apic/Getty Images

p50: Patrick Landmann/Getty images; De Agostini/Getty Images; Gamma-Keystone via Getty Images; New York Times Co./Getty images; Neal Grundy; Housewife/Getty Images; ssuaphoto/istock; Apic/Getty Images

p51: The Advertising Archives; Guerlain; The Advertising Archives; The Advertising Archives; Neal Grundy; Neal Grundy

p52–53 (map): Alice Tait

p52 (left to right): Sanjeri/istock; kira_an/istock; luknaja/istock

p53 (clockwise from top): Angela Conrady/Getty Images; Laitr Keiows/Shutterstock; felinda/istock; slallison/istock; phetphu/istock; marilyna/istock; rimglow/istock; dtimiraos/istock;